POCKET GUIDE
TO BREAST CANCER

Third Edition

Jones and Bartlett Series in Oncology

Jones and Bartlett Series in Oncology (continued)

POCKET GUIDE TO BREAST CANCER

Third Edition

Edited by

KAREN HASSEY DOW, PhD, RN, FAAN
Professor
School of Nursing, College of Health and Public Affairs
University of Central Florida
Orlando, Florida

JONES AND BARTLETT PUBLISHERS
Sudbury, Massachusetts
BOSTON   TORONTO   LONDON   SINGAPORE

World Headquarters
Jones and Bartlett Publishers
40 Tall Pine Drive
Sudbury, MA 01776
978–443–5000
www.jbpub.com
info@jbpub.com

Jones and Bartlett Publishers Canada
2406 Nikanna Road
Mississauga, ON L5C 2W6
CANADA

Jones and Bartlett Publishers International
Barb House, Barb Mews
London W6 7PA
UK

ISBN 0-7637-2995-7

Jones and Bartlett's books and products are available through most bookstores and online booksellers. To contact Jones and Bartlett Publishers directly, call 800-832-0034, fax 978-443-8000, or visit our website www.jbpub.com.

Substantial discounts on bulk quantities of Jones and Bartlett's publications are available to corporations, professional associations, and other qualified organizations. For details and specific discount information, contact the special sales department at Jones and Bartlett via the above contact information or send an email to specialsales@jbpub.com.

Production Credits
Acquisitions Editor: Kevin Sullivan
Associate Editor: Amy Sibley
Production Director: Amy Rose
Associate Production Editor: Renée Sekerak
Production Assistant: Rachel Rossi
Marketing Manager: Emily Ekle
Manufacturing and Inventory Coordinator: Amy Bacus
Manufacturing Buyer: Therese Bräuer
Design and Composition: Paw Print Media
Printing and Binding: United Graphics, Inc.

Printed in the United States of America
09 08 07 06 05   10 9 8 7 6 5 4 3 2 1

With love and appreciation for my mother Leonina and in loving memory of my father Orlando

Contents

Preface

Welcome to the third edition of the *Pocket Guide*. This edition is similar to the previous editions, with the goal of providing an easy-to-use, day-to-day reference for nurses caring for patients with breast cancer and their families. Similar to the first and second editions, the content of the pocket guide is divided into four parts: Epidemiology of Breast Cancer; Management of Primary Breast Cancer; Treatment of Recurrent Breast Cancer; and Quality-of-Life Issues in Breast Cancer. The chapters have been expanded and updated to provide the reader with current information. Two additional chapters have been added: Endocrine Therapy in Recurrent Disease and End-of-Life and Palliative Care. The reader should keep in mind that breast cancer care continues to undergo rapid developments and changes. Individual, programmatic, and institutional differences in the care of patients with breast cancer will vary.

Acknowledgment

Thanks to Sharon Austin for her assistance in manuscript preparation.

Disclaimer

Given the tremendous breakthroughs in cancer research and changes in clinical practice, the nature of breast cancer care is constantly evolving. Because science is constantly changing and research influences practice, the information contained in this book can be viewed as current at the time of publication. The information about drug dosages presented in this pocket guide is in accord with recommendations at the time of publication. However, before administering any drug, the reader is advised to check the manufacturer's product information sheet for the most current recommendations on dosage, precautions, and contraindications. The reader is advised that the authors, editor, reviewers, and publisher cannot be responsible for any errors or omissions in this handbook or for any consequences arising therefrom.

PART I

Epidemiology of Breast Cancer

CHAPTER ONE

Incidence, Epidemiology, and Survival

Trends in Incidence

- Breast cancer is the most common cancer in women in the United States (Cancer Statistics, 2005).

- The American Cancer Society (ACS) estimated 215,990 new cases of breast cancer in 2004.

- Breast cancer accounts for 32% of new cancer cases in American women (ACS, Cancer Statistics).

- The overall case rate per 100,000 age-adjusted women is about 118.4 for whites and 103.0 for blacks.

- Worldwide, 1.05 million new cases of cancer are projected (Parkin, 2004).

- The lifetime probability risk of developing breast cancer is one in seven (Cancer Statistics, 2004).

Survival

- Based on the National Cancer Institute's Surveillance, Epidemiology, and End Results (SEER) program, the 5-year relative survival rate for all women with localized invasive breast cancer is 96.5% (Ries, et al., 2004).

- The 5-year relative survival for female breast cancer is 88% for whites and 74% for blacks.

- The 5-year survival for all stages is 87% (from 1992–1999).

- Survival decreases with advanced stage of disease at diagnosis.

- Figure 1-1 shows the cancer incidence rates by race and ethnicity.

Mortality

- The ACS estimated 40,110 deaths due to breast cancer in 2004.

- Breast cancer is the second leading cause of cancer deaths in American women after lung cancer.

- It is the leading cause of cancer death in women age 40 to 55.

- It accounts for 15% of all cancer deaths in American women.

- Breast cancer deaths have declined since 1990.

Figure 1-1

Cancer Incidence Rates* by Race and Ethnicity, 1996–2000

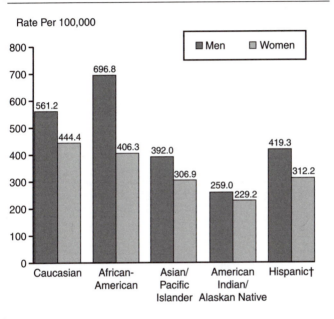

*Age-adjusted to the 2000 U.S. standard population.
†Hispanic is not mutually exclusive from Caucasians,
   African-Americans, Asian/Pacific Islanders, and American Indians.
Source: Surveillance, Epidemiology, and End Results Program,
   1975–2000, Division of Cancer Control and
   Population Sciences, National Cancer Institute, 2003.

- Factors relating to decreased mortality (Ries, et al., 2004):

  Mammographic screening

  Advances in systemic therapy

  Improved understanding of the mechanisms of recurrence and metastasis

- Table 1-1 shows 10-year survival by stage of disease.

TABLE 1-1
10-Year Survival by Stage

Stage	10-Year Survival (%)
0	95
I	88
II	66
III	36
IV	7

Source: Fremgen, et al., 1999.

- The highest decrease in mortality occurred in white and younger women (Ries, et al., 2004).
- Worldwide, there was a 1% to 2% reduction in mortality in countries having a high incidence. This includes the United States, Canada, and the United Kingdom (Mettlin, 1999).

Racial and Ethnic Differences (ACS, Cancer Statistics, 2004)

- Incidence and mortality rates vary by race and ethnicity.

- Caucasian women have the highest incidence rates followed by African-Americans, Hispanics, Asian-Pacific Islanders, and American Indian/Alaskan native women.

- African-American women have a higher death rate from breast cancer, compared with any other racial or ethnic group.

- African-American women have a poorer probability of survival once they are diagnosed.

- Factors associated with higher mortality in African-American women include:

  Later stage at diagnosis

  Disease characteristics such as larger tumor size, greater nodal involvement, estrogen receptor (ER)—negative tumors, shorter time to recurrence

  Unequal access to care

- Table 1-2 shows the incidence and mortality by racial and ethnic groups.

TABLE 1-2

Incidence and Mortality Rates by Race and Ethnicity, United States: 1996–2000

Racial/Ethnic Group	Incidence	Mortality
White	114.0	25.3
Black	100.2	31.4
Asian/Pacific Islander	74.6	11.2
Native American	33.4	12.1
Hispanic	68.9	15.1

Source: Cancer Statistics, 2004.

REFERENCES

American Cancer Society. (2005). Cancer Statistics, 2005. Retrieved May 4, 2005, from www.cancer.org/docroot/PRO/content/ PRO_1_1_1_Cancer_Statistics_2005_Presentation.asp

American Cancer Society. (2004). Cancer Statistics. (2004). Retrieved October 20, 2004, from www.cancer.org/downloads

Fremgen, A., Bland, K., McGinnis, L. J., & et al. (1999). Clinical highlights from the National Cancer Data Base, 1999. *A Cancer Journal for Clinicians, 49*, 145–158.

Mettlin, C. (1999). Global breast cancer mortality statistics. *CA: A Cancer Journal for Clinicians, 49*, 138–144.

Parkin, D. (2004). International variation. *Oncogene, 23*, 6329–6340.

Ries, L., Eisner, M. P., Kosary, C. L., Hankey, B. F., Miller, B. A., Clegg, L., et al. (2004). SEER Cancer Statistics Review, 1975–2001, National Cancer Institute, from http://seer.cancer.gov/csr/1975_2001/

CHAPTER TWO

Nongenetic Risk Factors and Inherited Predisposition

Background (Clark, 2004)

- Risk factors, both nongenetic and inherited predisposition, are of concern and a source of confusion among women.
- About 90–95% of all breast cancers are sporadic, with about 5–10% inherited.

Major Risk Factors (Willett, et al., 2004)

- Female gender

  Breast cancer occurs predominately among females.

  Breast cancer is rare among men with about 1,500 new cases annually.

- Advancing age

> *Breast cancer is rare among women younger than age 20 years.*
>
> *Incidence increases with age, with a large increase by age 50.*
>
> *Risk is 1 in 39 before age 50.*
>
> *Risk is 1 in 29 before age 60.*
>
> *Lifetime risk is 1 in 7.*

- Family history of breast cancer

  Increased risk when breast cancer occurs in first-degree relative (i.e., mother, sister, or daughter)

- Benign proliferative disease

  Atypical hyperplasia

  1. Women with atypical hyperplasia are more likely to develop breast cancer.

  2. The risk may decrease after menopause.

  Lobular carcinoma in situ (LCIS)

  1. LCIS is considered a marker or risk factor rather than a precursor to breast cancer.

  2. Women with LCIS have an increased risk of 1% per year for developing breast cancer.

  3. The lesion is usually asymptomatic, incidental microscopic finding that does not show as a mass on mammography.

  4. It is seen more often in younger than older women.

Reproductive Risk Factors (Willett, et al., 2004)

- Age at menarche:

    Earlier age at menarche increases risk.

    Shorter menstrual cycles are associated with increased risk.

    Long and irregular cycles are associated with reduced breast cancer risk.

    Early menarche and late menopause are related to increased total lifetime number of menstrual cycles, with a corresponding increase in breast cancer risk.

    Long exposure to estrogen with uninterrupted menstrual cycles is thought to be a mechanism for increased risk.

- Nulliparity is an increased risk, compared with parity.

- Younger age at first full-term pregnancy associated with lower risk.

- Higher number of births associated with lower risk.

- Age at menopause:

    Late menopause after age 55 increases risk.

    Women having bilateral oophorectomy before age 45 have lower risk compared with women having natural menopause.

    Later age at menopause associated with increased risk.

    Reduction in risk with early menopause is likely a result of the cessation of breast cell division and a decrease in endogenous hormone levels.

- Prenatal exposure to estrogen.

  Strong inverse relationship between preeclampsia during pregnancy and decreased risk of breast cancer.

- Induced abortion.

  Current evidence does not support a relationship between induced abortion and increased risk.

Exogenous Hormone Risk Factors (Willett, et al., 2004)

- Meta-analyses of studies of women who had used oral contraceptives did not show an association with breast cancer risk.
- Young women who use oral contraceptives for a long period of time have an increased risk.
- Hormone replacement therapy (HRT) of long duration is associated with increased risk.

Energy Expenditure as Risk Factors

- Weight gain

  High-energy intake that accelerates growth and earlier menstruation in childhood and weight gain in middle life increase the risk of breast cancer.

Dietary Risk Factors

- Dietary fat has not been associated with increased risk.
- Alcohol intake of more than two drinks per day increases risk.

- Dietary fiber; micronutrients, including vitamins E and C; and selenium do not support a protective factor from breast cancer.

- There may be a modest protective effect of vitamin A from breast cancer.

- Phytoestrogens in soy products may have a promising potential to decrease risk.

- Caffeine intake through drinking coffee or tea does not demonstrate an increased risk of breast cancer.

Environmental Risk Factors

- Radiation therapy delivered as treatment at a young age.

  Young women exposed to ionizing radiation to the chest at a young age for treatment of Hodgkin's disease have an increased risk of breast cancer.

- Electromagnetic field exposure (EMF) and breast cancer risk are weak.

- Environmental exposure to pesticides and organochlorines does not appear to be a risk factor in the development of breast cancer.

Breast Cancer Risk Assessment

- The Breast Cancer Risk Assessment Tool is an Internet tool to project a woman's individualized estimate for invasive breast cancer over a 5-year period and over her lifetime.

- The tool can be used as part of discussion about a woman's risk.

- The tool underestimates the risk for women with breast cancer and does not take into account the specific genetic mutations in BRCA1 or BRCA2.

- Risk projections assume that women are receiving regular breast examinations and screening mammograms.

- Factors used in determining risk include:

  Age

  Age at menarche

  Age at first live birth

  Number of first-degree relatives (i.e. mother, sisters, and/or daughters) with breast cancer

  Number of previous breast positive or negative breast biopsies

  Biopsy with atypical hyperplasia

- Risk factors *not* used in determining risk include:

  Menopause

  Tissue density on mammogram

  Contraceptive use

  Hormone therapy use

  High dietary fat

  Level of physical activity

  Obesity

  Environmental exposure

- The Breast Cancer Risk Assessment Tool can be accessed online at http://brca.nci.nih.gov/brc/q1.htm

Inherited Breast Cancer Predisposition
(Domchek & Weber, 2004)

- Mutations in breast cancer susceptibility genes are responsible for 5% to 10% of all breast cancers.

- Mutations in single cancer susceptibility genes are associated with increased susceptibility to breast and ovarian cancer.

- Inherited breast cancers comprise 5% to 10% of all breast cancers.

- Inherited predisposition is autosomal dominant.

- Individuals who carry the mutation have increased risk up to 50% of developing breast cancer.

- Hereditary breast cancer is characterized by:

   Early age at onset (about 5 to 15 years before sporadic breast cancer)

   Bilateral breast cancer

   Vertical transmission from either mother or father

   Association with other cancers including ovarian and prostate cancers

- There are two types of genetic damage responsible for the development of the malignant phenotype:

   Activation of proto-oncogenes

   Inactivation of tumor-suppressor genes

> *Mutated tumor-suppressor genes lose critical functions in regulating the cell cycle, cellular response to DNA damage and preventing the mutation of other critical genes.*

- Presence of gene mutation BRCA1 or BRCA2

  Inherited gene mutation occurs in 1 in 200 women.

  Inherited gene mutation occurs in 1 in 40 women of Eastern European descent.

  Gene mutation can be inherited from either parent.

  BRCA1 mutation increases the chance of breast cancer between 35% to 85%. BRCA2 mutation increases the chance of breast cancer from 20% to 60%.

BRCA1

- BRCA1 is located on chromosome 17q21, and this mutation is associated with early-onset breast cancer.
- BRCA1 is thought to be a tumor-suppressor gene.
- BRCA1 is associated with an increased risk of ovarian cancer.
- BRCA1 tumors tend to have aggressive pathologic features, such as high nuclear grade and are often estrogen-receptor negative and progesterone-receptor negative.

BRCA2

- Mutations may contribute to fewer cases of early-onset breast cancer, compared with BRCA1.
- BRCA2 is thought to be a tumor-suppressor gene.
- BRCA2 mutations are associated with an elevated risk for the development of other cancers, such as ovarian, prostate, and pancreatic cancer.
- BRCA2 mutations are associated with a 6% lifetime risk of male breast cancer.

Characteristics Associated with the Likelihood of BRCA1 or BRCA2 Mutation

- Early onset breast cancer
- Bilateral breast cancer
- Personal history of breast and ovarian cancer
- Breast cancer in one or more male family members

Characteristics Associated with the Likelihood of BRCA1 Mutation

- Multiple cases of familial breast cancer
- Familial presence of breast and ovarian cancers
- One or more family members with two primary cancers
- Having Ashkenazi Jewish family background

Other Inherited Breast Cancer Predispositions
(Clark, 2004; Strauss-Trainin, 1996)

Li-Fraumeni Syndrome

- Autosomal dominant disorder associated with the increased risk of several tumors, including soft-tissue sarcomas, breast cancer, osteosarcoma, adrenocortical carcinoma, brain tumors, acute leukemia, and possibly other cancers.

- Fifty percent of patients have germline mutations that fall within a single small region on the *p53* tumor-suppressor gene.

- About 50% of women with the Li-Fraumeni Syndrome may develop breast cancer. This disorder probably affects less than 1% of all breast cancer cases.

Ataxia-Telangiectasia (AT)

- Autosomal recessive disorder characterized by the development of cerebellar ataxia, telangiectases, immune defects, predisposition to malignancy, and hypersensitivity to ionizing radiation.

- Affected individuals have a 10% to 20% risk of developing cancer, especially lymphomas and lymphocytic leukemias, but also epithelial tumors, including breast cancer.

- Relatives of individuals with ataxia-telangiectasia appear to have an increased risk of breast cancer.

Muir-Torre Syndrome

- Rare autosomal dominant condition that includes multiple benign sebaceous adenomas and carcinomas, basal and squamous cell carcinomas, and keratoacanthomas of the skin, as well as multiple internal malignancies.

- Inherited cancers include tumors of the colon, stomach, esophagus, breast, uterus, ovaries, bladder, and larynx, as well as squamous cell carcinoma of the mucous membranes.

Cowden's Syndrome

- Autosomal dominant trait is characterized by multiple hamartomatous lesions of skin, mucous membranes, breast, and thyroid.

- Fifty percent of affected females have fibrocystic disease of the breast as well as breast cancer, of which 33% are bilateral breast cancer.

- Increased incidence of cancers of the thyroid, colon, uterus, cervix, lung, bladder, skin, and lymphoreticular system exists.

Peutz-Jeghers Syndrome

- Early onset autosomal dominant disorder is characterized by the association of black or bluish melanin spots on the lips, perioral region, buccal mucosa,

hands, arms, feet, and legs, with gastrointestinal polyposis.
- Syndrome carries increased risk of cancers of the breast, GI tract, and ovarian sex cord.

Genetic Testing and Risk Counseling (Cummings & Olopade, 1998; Metcalfe, et al., 2000)

- Genetic testing for BRCA1 and BRCA2 available since 1996.
- Factors that influence individuals to proceed with genetic testing:

    Cost of genetic testing

    Additional benefit from knowing results of genetic testing

    Whether results of genetic testing will influence clinical decision making

    Personal estimate of inherited risk

    Health beliefs

- Risk counseling

    Conduct evaluation of family history for at least two generations.

    Predisposition testing is helpful when family member with breast cancer undergoes the initial testing.

    Age, education, and previous diagnosis of cancer are important aspects in decision making after positive genetic testing.

Elements of informed consent must be considered for an individual considering testing for cancer susceptibility. They include:

1. Information about the tests, risks, benefits, and efficacy
2. Option of risk estimation without genetic testing
3. Risk of passing a mutation to the next generation
4. Technical accuracy (sensitivity and specificity) of testing
5. Options for management strategies for carriers include:
   - making decisions about the nature, frequency, and screening and surveillance procedures
   - chemoprevention
   - risk-reducing surgery
6. Psychosocial risks and distress
7. Potential for work-related discrimination
8. Costs of testing and counseling

Breast cancer risk assessment is ideally done by using a multidisciplinary approach.

- Management

  Close surveillance, education, and counseling are important.

  Prophylactic mastectomy may be considered as an option.

REFERENCES

Clark, P. M. (2004). Nongenetic and heritable risk factors. In K. H. Dow (Ed.), *Contemporary issues in breast cancer: A nursing perspective* (2nd ed., pp. 10–24). Sudbury, MA: Jones & Bartlett.

Cummings, S., & Olopade, O. (1998). Predisposition testing for inherited breast cancer. *Oncology, 12*(8), 1227–1241; discussion 1241–1222.

Domchek, S., & Weber, B. (2004). Inherited genetic factors and breast cancer. In J. R. Harris, M. Lippman, M. Morrow, & C. K. Osborne (Eds.), *Diseases of the breast* (3rd ed., pp. 277–302). Philadelphia: Lippincott Williams & Wilkins.

Metcalfe, K., Liede, A., Hoodfar, E., & et al. (2000). An evaluation of needs of female BRCA1 and BRCA2 carriers undergoing genetic counseling. *Journal of Medical Genetics, 37*, 866–874.

Strauss-Trainin, A. (1996). Genetics and breast cancer risk. In K. H. Dow (Ed.), *Contemporary issues in breast cancer* (pp. 3–19). Sudbury, MA: Jones and Bartlett.

Willett, W., Rockhill, B., Hankinson, S., & et al. (2004). Nongenetic factors in the causation of breast cancer. In J. R. Harris, M. Lippman, M. Morrow, & C. K. Osborne (Eds.), *Diseases of the breast* (3rd ed., pp. 221–276). Philadelphia: Lippincott Williams & Wilkins.

CHAPTER THREE

Prevention Strategies

Introduction

- There has been an increased attention to prevention of breast cancer in recent years.

- Various prevention strategies may be used based on a woman's level of risk.

- Although there are several nonmodifiable risk factors such as family history of breast cancer, there is increased attention to modifiable risk factors such as lifestyle changes.

- Although selected women at high risk may be candidates for chemoprevention or risk-reducing surgery, all women can practice lifestyle modification.

- Table 3-1 summarizes the scientific beliefs of known and unknown factors in breast cancer prevention.

TABLE 3-1

Scientific Beliefs of Known and Unknown Factors in Breast Cancer Prevention

Concept	Unknown
1. Cancer development likely due to molecular step-by-step progression of changes to breast cells leading to breast cancer.	Exact biologic mechanisms
2. Cancer development from carcinogenic exposures can take years to develop.	All environmental factors that may promote breast cancer
3. Wide range international variation in breast cancer rates suggest breast cancer may be preventable by modifying lifestyle and environmental determinants.	Mechanisms of interaction of genetic, environmental, and lifestyle factors
4. Cancer development can be reversible.	Timing and interventions to reverse breast cancer development
5. Deleterious mutations in certain genes can lead to a high risk of breast cancer.	All possible genetic mutations that lead to an increased risk
6. Cancer development is likely due to the interaction of genetic hormonal, lifestyle, and environmental factors.	Interaction and timing of factors

- Table 3-2 summarizes factors that are implicated in breast cancer development and possible preventive actions that can be taken.

TABLE 3-2

Summary of Factors Implicated in Breast Cancer Development and Possible Preventive Actions

Factor	Possible Preventive Actions
Environmental	
Irradiation exposure causing germline and/or somatic breast cell mutations in developing fetus and individuals	Avoidance of irradiation, particularly in utero and between menarche and first full-term pregancy
	Early screening of women who had mantle radiation for Hodgkin's Disease
Genetic	
Germline mutations in BRCA1/2; p53; pTEN	Genetic screening/counseling and current breast cancer prevention options of increased surveillance, chemoprevention, preventive surgery
Limited repair of acquired breast epithelial cell DNA damage (ATM)	Limit exposure to irradiation and cigarette smoke
Hormonal	
Increased estrogen exposure/prolonged duration of ovulation	Delay onset of menarche
	Initiate early menopause
	Oophorectomy; LHRH agonists
	Avoid delayed childbearing

(continues)

TABLE 3-2 (*continued*)
Summary of Factors Implicated in Breast Cancer Development and Possible Preventive Actions

Factor	Possible Preventive Actions
	Reduce ovarian activity (prolonged lactation)
	Modify endogenous hormone levels
	Exercise, avoid weight gain; limit alcohol
	Low-fat diet
	Aromatase inhibitors
	Avoid exogenous hormones
	Modify hormone receptor function
	Selective estrogen receptor modulators: tamoxifen, raloxifene, phytoestrogens
	Modify estrogen metabolism
	Modify breast growth factor action

Approaches to Prevention (Bucholtz, 2004)

- After breast cancer risk assessment, different levels of risk vary from average risk to increased risk to high risk based on family history suggesting genetic predisposition.

- Figure 3-1 shows differential breast cancer prevention strategies based on breast cancer risk.

- Prevention approaches include:

  General screening and lifestyle modification for women of low to average risk

  Chemoprevention, preventive surgery for women of increased risk

  Chemoprevention, preventive surgery, and genetic counseling for women at higher risk with genetic predisposition.

Chemoprevention

- *Chemoprevention* is the use of a drug to reduce cancer risk.

- Two chemoprevention trials include the BCPT and STAR (see pp. 29–31).

- Breast Cancer Prevention Trial (BCPT) P-1 (Fisher, et al., 1998)

  The BCPT was a randomized clinical trial evaluating whether tamoxifen can prevent breast cancer in women at increased risk of developing the disease.

FIGURE 3-1

Suggested Breast Cancer Prevention Strategies Based on Breast Cancer Risk

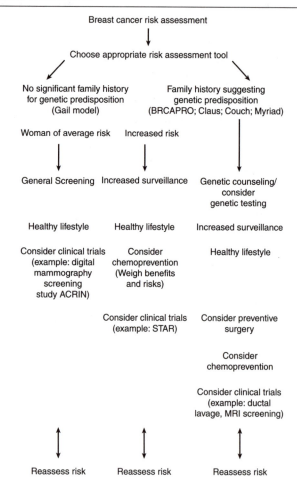

*BCPT looked at whether tamoxifen decreased the number of
heart attacks and reduced the number of bone fractures. It concluded tamoxifen works against breast
cancer by interfering with estrogen activity. Tamoxifen
stops or slows down the growth of cancer cells.*

*BCPT recruited participants from 1992 to 1997 and
enrolled over 13,000 women 35 years and older
across 300 centers in the United States and Canada.*

BCPT was funded by the National Cancer Institute (NCI).

*Women at increased risk were eligible to participate in
BCPT*

1. Women 60 years of age and older qualified
   based on age alone.

2. Women age 35 to 59 with an increased risk
   of breast cancer equivalent to women age 60
   years were also eligible to participate. About
   40% of the women who participated were in
   this age group.

3. Women with lobular carcinoma in situ were
   eligible based on the diagnosis alone.

Factors identified in risk calculation included:

1. Number of first-degree relatives (i.e.,
   mother, daughters, sisters) diagnosed with
   breast cancer

2. Parity and age at first delivery

3. Number of breast biopsies particularly atypical hyperplasia

4.   Age at first menstrual period

Minority participation was 4% and included blacks, Asians, and Hispanics.

Results showed a 45% reduction in breast cancer incidence among high-risk participants.

Young women who met the criteria and took tamoxifen had no benefit and had increased side effects.

Tamoxifen is contraindicated in women during pregnancy because animal research suggests deleterious effect in utero.

Women age 35 to 49 who took tamoxifen had increased risk for endometrial cancer and deep vein thrombosis similar to those taking the placebo.

Women age 50 and older had four times the chance of developing endometrial cancer and three times the chance for developing deep vein thrombosis and pulmonary embolism.

Tamoxifen use in BCPT showed a 2.5 increase in the risk of endometrial cancer overall.

For more information about BCPT access www.nsabp.pitt.edu/BCPT_Q&A.pdf (National Surgical Adjuvant Breast & Bowel Project, NSABP, 2004a).

- BCPT Results

  Over 13,000 women at increased risk (i.e., at least 60 years of age or 35 to 59 years with predicted risk of at least 1.7 on Breast Cancer Risk Assessment) received either tamoxifen 20 mg daily or placebo for 5 years.

Risk of invasive breast cancer reduced by 49% in women age 35 and older.

Women with atypical hyperplasia had an 86% reduction in risk.

Tamoxifen did not affect the incidence of estrogen receptor (ER)–negative tumors.

Women with lobular carcinoma in situ (LCIS) had a 56% reduction in risk.

Beneficial effects of tamoxifen included a reduction in hip, radius, and spine fractures.

Conclusion: Tamoxifen decreased the incidence of invasive and noninvasive breast cancer and is an appropriate preventive agent in women at increased risk.

Tamoxifen is approved in the United States for reduction of breast cancer risk in women at high risk.

Tamoxifen therapy lasts for 5 years, and, thus, risk reduction must be weighed against potential risks of long-term drug usage (Gail, et al., 1999).

- Chemoprevention: Study of Raloxifene and Tamoxifen

    The Study of Tamoxifen and Raloxifene (STAR) is a large breast cancer prevention trial.

    STAR compares tamoxifen, a drug known to reduce the chance of developing breast cancer with raloxifene, a drug that has the potential to reduce risk of breast cancer.

    Participants receive either tamoxifen or raloxifene for 5 years.

STAR is a randomized double-blind clinical trial including 19,000 postmenopausal women at high risk for breast cancer.

Breast cancer risk is calculated based on a woman's age, family history of breast cancer, and personal medical history.

Raloxifene is FDA approved for prevention and treatment of osteoporosis in post-menopausal women.

Tamoxifen and raloxifene are in a class of agents called selective estrogen receptor modulators (SERM)*.*

Both tamoxifen and raloxifene have common side effects including hot flashes and vaginal discharge.

One serious side effect from raloxifene is blood clots.

Women who are not eligible to participate in STAR include women with a history of cancer, blood clots, stroke, irregular heartbeats, high blood pressure, and uncontrolled diabetes.

For more information about tamoxifen, raloxifene and breast cancer access www.cancer.gov/cancertopics/ understandingcancer/estrogenreceptors. This is a tutorial that explains estrogen receptors, tamoxifen, and raloxifene (NCI, 2004b).

For more information about STAR access www.nsabp.pitt.edu/STAR/Index.html (NSABP, 2004b).

For more information about cancer clinical trials access www.cancer.gov/clinical_trials/ (NCI, 2004a).

Preventive Surgery

- Preventive or prophylactic mastectomy is the surgical removal of one or both breasts to prevent or reduce the risk of breast cancer in high-risk women.

- First reported retrospective study to demonstrate benefits of bilateral preventive mastectomy in women at increased risk (Hartmann, et al., 1999).

- Potential candidates for preventive mastectomy:

  Personal history of breast cancer

  Strong family or personal history of breast cancer

  Multiple previous breast biopsies

  Diagnosis of LCIS or atypical hyperplasia

  Inherited genetic susceptibility

- Benefits include satisfaction with decision to have surgery and reduce risk of breast cancer.

- Complications of preventive mastectomy include:

  Chest numbness

  Absent nipple sensation

  Seromas, hematomas

  Pain

  Dissatisfaction with cosmetic results

  Potential psychological trauma.

- Nurse's role in preventive mastectomy (Gross, 2000)

  Facilitate the referral to a plastic surgeon to evaluate reconstructive options.

> *Explore the potential psychological and social effects of prophylactic and bilateral mastectomy.*
>
> *Educate the patient about the surgical procedure and potential complications, including bleeding, infection, and flap reconstruction loss.*

- Preventive oophorectomy has been considered in women who are BRCA mutation carriers to prevent ovarian cancer.
- There are currently no available data to define the magnitude of reduction of breast cancer risk (Bucholtz, 2004).
- Potential risks include surgical risk and early menopause.

Lifestyle Modification

- Lifestyle modification can be practiced by all women to reduce breast cancer risk.
- Breast cancer risk may be reduced by lifestyle modification such as:

  Weight control and weight reduction

  Smoking cessation

  Decreased alcohol consumption

  Exercise

Weight, Weight Gain, and Adiposity

- Weight gain is a modifiable risk factor to help reduce breast cancer risk.

- Obesity and hormone replacement therapy (HRT) are associated with an increased risk of breast cancer in postmenopausal women (Feigelson, et al., 2003).

- After menopause, estradiol is produced through the conversion of androgens to estrogens in fat tissue.

- In premenopausal women, high body weight is associated with a reduced risk of breast cancer because obesity leads to irregular menstrual cycles and fewer ovulatory cycles.

- Feigelson and associates (2004) found that weight gain is a stronger predictor of breast cancer risk compared with body mass index (BMI) among non-HRT users. There is an observed twofold increased risk among women who gain 60 pounds or more. Among HRT users, there is a higher rate of breast cancer, but no increased risk associated with weight gain.

- In the United States, there has been a steady increase in obesity since the 1960s. However, since the 1980s, there has been a staggering increase in obesity with related diseases.

- Excess adiposity or obesity may be responsible for up to 25% of breast cancers. Thus, the critical importance of minimizing weight gain throughout one's lifetime (Petrelli, et al., 2002).

- Data from the National Weight Control Registry (see www.uchsc.edu/nutrition/WyattJortberg/nwcr.htm) of adults who have had more than 30 pound weight loss and kept the weight loss for over a year have used the following strategies to maintain weight loss:

Frequent self-monitoring of weight and food intake

High levels of regular physical activity.

Smoking Cessation

- Smoking increases the risk of lung and other cancers and increases the risk of heart disease.
- Smoking affects one's overall health but has not had a direct effect on the development of breast cancer (Hamajima, et al., 2002).

Alcohol Consumption

- Moderate to high amounts of alcohol consumption have been associated with increased breast cancer incidence (Hamajima, et al., 2002; Smith-Warner, et al., 1998).
- Relative risk increases by 10% in women who consume one alcoholic drink a day compared with nondrinkers.
- Ethanol may increase the risk because it induces increased levels of circulating estrogens and depletes folate.
- Women at low to moderate risk may consider decreasing risk of breast cancer through reduction in alcohol consumption.

Exercise

- Exercise may reduce the risk of breast cancer by reducing hormonal levels.

- Decreased risk of breast cancer may be associated with increasing lifetime physical activity (Bernstein, et al., 1994).

- Potential public health benefit with a modifiable risk factor such as exercise can decrease breast cancer risk (Thune, et al., 1997).

REFERENCES

Bernstein, L., Henderson, B., Hanisch, R., et al. (1994). Physical exercise and reduced risk of breast cancer in young women. *Journal of the National Cancer Institute, 86*, 1403–1408.

Bucholtz, J. (2004). Prevention strategies. In K. H. Dow (Ed.), *Contemporary issues in breast cancer: A nursing perspective* (2nd ed., pp. 25–44). Sudbury, MA: Jones & Bartlett.

Feigelson, H. S., Jonas, C. R., Robertson, A. S., McCullough, M. L., Thun, M. J., & Calle, E. E. (2003). Alcohol, folate, methionine, and risk of incident breast cancer in the American Cancer Society Cancer Prevention Study II Nutrition Cohort. *Cancer Epidemiology and Biomarkers Prevention, 12*(2), 161–164.

Feigelson, H. S., Jonas, C. R., Teras, L. R., Thun, M. J., & Calle, E. E. (2004). Weight gain, body mass index, hormone replacement therapy, and postmenopausal breast cancer in a large prospective study. *Cancer Epidemiology Biomarkers & Prevention, 13*(2), 220–224.

Fisher, B., Costantino, J., Wickerham, D., et al. (1998). Tamoxifen for prevention of breast cancer: Report of the National Surgical Adjuvant Breast and Bowel Project P-1 Study. *Journal of the National Cancer Institute, 16,* 1381–1388.

Gail, M., Costantino, J., Bryant, J., et al. (1999). Weighing the risks and benefits of tamoxifen treatment for preventing breast cancer. *Journal of the National Cancer Institute, 91,* 1829–1846.

Gross, R. (2000). Breast cancer: Risk factors, screening, and prevention. *Seminars in Oncology Nursing, 16,* 176–184.

Hamajima, N., Hirose, K., Tajima, K., Rohan, T., Calle, E. E., Heath, C. W., Jr., et al. (2002). Alcohol, tobacco and breast cancer—Collaborative reanalysis of individual data from 53 epidemiological studies, including 58,515 women with breast cancer and 95,067 women without the disease. *British Journal of Cancer, 87*(11), 1234–1245.

Hartmann, L., Schaid, D., & Woods, J. (1999). Efficacy of bilateral prophylactic mastectomy in women with a family history of breast cancer. *New England Journal of Medicine, 340,* 77–84.

National Cancer Institute. (2004a). *Clinical trials.* Retrieved October 18, 2004, from www.cancer.gov/clinical_trials

National Cancer Institute. (2004b). *Understanding Estrogen Receptors, Tamoxifen, and Raloxifene.* Retrieved October 20, 2004, from http://press2.nci.nih.gov/sciencebehind/estrogen/estrogen01.htm

National Surgical Adjuvant Breast & Bowel Project (NSABP). (2004a). *Breast cancer prevention trial.* Retrieved October 19, 2004, from www.nsabp.pitt.edu/BCPT_Q&A.pdf

National Surgical Adjuvant Breast & Bowel Project (NSABP). (2004b). *Study of tamoxifen and raloxifene.* Retrieved October 18, 2004, from www.nsabp.pitt.edu/STAR/Index.html

Petrelli, J. M., Calle, E. E., Rodriguez, C., & Thun, M. J. (2002). Body mass index, height, and postmenopausal breast cancer mortality in a prospective cohort of U.S. women. *Cancer Causes Control, 13*(4), 325–332.

Smith-Warner, S., Spiegelman, D., Yaunn, S., et al. (1998). Alcohol and breast cancer in women: A pooled analysis of cohort studies. *Journal of the American Medical Association, 279*, 535–540.

Thune, I., Brenn, T., Lund, E., et al. (1997). Physical activity and the risk of breast cancer. *New England Journal of Medicine, 336*, 1269–1275.

CHAPTER FOUR

Screening and Early Detection

Principles of Cancer Screening
   (Smith & D'Orsi, 2004)

- Screening distinguishes among individuals who are likely and not likely to have a disease.
- Criteria for screening
  1. Disease must be an important health problem.
  2. Disease must be in the period when the disease is detectable in an asymptomatic individual.
  3. Screening test must be effective, accurate, and affordable.

Goals of Breast Cancer Screening

- Earlier diagnosis in asymptomatic individuals
- Reduction in mortality due to early detection

Triad of Screening Methods (Machia, 2004)

- Triad of screening methods is mammography, clinical breast examination (CBE), and breast self-examination (BSE).

- Current guidelines for breast cancer screening vary among various organizations. Table 4-1 shows the different guidelines for breast cancer screening of average-risk asymptomatic women.

Screening Mammography

- Screening mammography is the most sensitive method for detecting early-stage breast cancer.

- Screening mammography may decrease mortality.

- NCI Statement on Mammography Screening can be accessed online at www.nci.nih.gov/newscenter/mammstatement31jan02 (NCI, 2004).

- Baseline mammogram

  Begin by age 40 and then every 1 to 2 years for average-risk asymptomatic women.

  Begin by age 25 for high-risk women or 5 years earlier than the earliest age when breast cancer was diagnosed in a family member.

  Initiate yearly mammography in women with an identified genetic predisposition (BRCA1 and BRCA2 mutations).

- Benefits (U.K. Trial, 1999; Hendrick, et al., 1997)

TABLE 4-1
Guidelines for Screening Average-Risk Asymptomatic Women

Screening Technique	American Cancer Society	National Cancer Institute	U.S. Preventive Services Task Force
Breast self-examination	Monthly starting age 20	No recommendation	Evidence is insufficient to make recommendation either for or against routine BSE alone.
Clinical breast examination (CBE)	20–39 years: Every 3 years Annually starting at age 40	No recommendation	Evidence is insufficient to make recommendation either for or against routine CBE alone.
Mammogram	Annually by age 40	Start by age 40 Conduct every 1 to 2 years for women who are at average risk Women at higher risk should consult physician about screening before age 40	Every 1 to 2 years for women age 40 and older.

Sources: Smith, R., von Eschenbach, A., Wender, R., et al., 2001; NCI, 1997; USPSTF, 2004.

Reduction in mortality by 17% in asymptomatic women age 40 to 49

Reduction in mortality by 25% to 30% in asymptomatic women age 50 to 69

Smaller reduction in mortality for women over age 75

Detection of nonpalpable lesions that are correlated with a better prognosis (20% to 30% of nonpalpable lesions malignant at biopsy)

Greater than 85% sensitivity with mammography

- Limitations

  Less effective in younger women due to breast tissue density

  Cannot differentiate benign from malignant lesions

- Barriers to mammographic screening

  Lack of recommendation by primary care physician

  False belief that having one mammogram is enough

  False belief that mammograms are not required in the absence of symptoms

  Underutilization pattern seen in older women and minorities

  Lack of insurance coverage and costs of mammography

  - Age at which women begin mammographic screening varies considerably. Colbert and colleagues (2004) found that the median age in which women had their first mammogram was 40.4 years. Sixty percent of women had first mammogram by the end of 40.9 years. Nearly 90% started screening by 50 years of age.

- ■ Women who began screening later included blacks, Hispanics, those who are obese, those without a primary care provider, those without private health insurance, and those who are non-English speaking (Colbert, et al., 2004).

- Patterns of use of annual screening are low (Blanchard, et al., 2004).

  Underutilization of return screening noted among underserved women, minority women, those who are socioeconomically disadvantaged, non-English speaking women, and women without private health insurance.

Clinical Breast Examination

- Recommended with every general physical examination.

- CBE every 3 years starting between age 20 to 39, according to the American Cancer Society (ACS)

- Annually by age 40 in conjunction with mammography

- One benefit of CBE is that it improves the detection of breast cancer by 5% to 20%.

- One limitation of CBE is that the accuracy depends on the experience and skill of the examiner.

Breast Self-Examination

- Begin by age 20 and continue monthly, according to the ACS.

- Benefits
    1. Helps increase breast health awareness.
    2. Provides women with the ability to understand their anatomy and the contour of their breasts. Women need adequate instruction in learning how to perform BSE properly.
    3. Is low cost and low risk.
- Limitations
    1. Anxiety and avoidance behaviors are associated with the performance of BSE.
    2. There is lower sensitivity in detecting breast cancer compared with mammography.
    3. BSE is complementary to mammography and should not replace it.

Other Screening Methods

- Search for methods to increase the accuracy of the screening and to overcome barriers relating to film-screen mammography.
- Types
    1. Digital mammography
    2. Magnetic resonance imaging (MRI)
    3. Positron emission tomography
    4. Breast duct lavage and needle aspiration
    5. Mammotome
    6. Ultrasound

Digital Mammography

- Digital processing is a computerized tool for capturing, enhancing, and storing mammographic images with the goal of increasing the accuracy of screening mammography, improving diagnosis, reducing the number of negative biopsies, and improving the continuity of care.

- The Food and Drug Administration (FDA) approved digital mammography.

- The process uses computer-aided digital displays and reduces the time from imaging to display.

- Digital images can be manipulated, with adjustments for contrast and brightness.

- Suspicious areas of concern can be magnified.

- Benefits (Smith & D'Orsi, 2004):

  Computer video diagnosis and computer-aided detection (CAD) may decrease false-positive screening rates.

  The process may be useful in imaging dense breast tissue.

  It decreases the time required for breast compression.

- Limitations:

  Digital images must be viewed on specialized monitors that are extremely expensive.

  The brightness of the specialized monitors is not equivalent to that of the traditional mammographic view box.

  Image manipulation may require more time for interpreting results.

  Full-field digital screening mammography units are costly.

Magnetic Resonance Imaging

- MRI is an imaging technique that does not involve radiation.

- There has been increased interest in MRI because it can overcome problems of lack of mammographic specificity.

- Contrast agents tailored for use with MRI have improved sensitivity and specificity.

- Contrast-enhanced imaging is based on the vascularity and vessel permeability difference between benign and malignant lesions.

  Benign conditions are poorly vascularized.

  Malignant lesions require vascular supplies.

- Specific use of MRI

  Potential for screening women at high genetic risk with BRCA1 or BRCA2 mutation

  Differentiates multifocal, multicentric, or diffuse masses

  Sensitive in detecting small lesions less than 1 cm in size

  May be used when patient has very dense breasts

- Benefits

  Able to detect occult tumors that are not detected using mammography or CBE

- Limitations

  Costly and invasive technique

  Must undergo quality assurance evaluation and standard setting similar to film-screen mammography

Positron Emission Tomography Scanning (Mautner, et al., 2000)

- Procedure is based on the knowledge that malignant tumors use more glucose than normal tissue.
- When glucose is trapped in tumor cells, it allows imaging by means of positron emission tomography.
- Process offers high specificity for malignancy.
- Sensitivity is limited to tumors less than 8 mm.
- Scanning has potential for screening women at high genetic risk.

Breast Duct Lavage and Nipple Aspiration

- Over 95% of breast cancers start in cells lining the inside of the milk ducts.
- Changes in the DNA of nipple aspirate, protein biomarkers, or patterns of proteins in nipple aspirate fluid may be a useful and early indicator of cancer (Fabian, et al., 2000; Sharma, et al., 2004).
- Methods of obtaining fluid from the milk ducts:
    1. Breast duct lavage involves cells from milk ducts in the breast that are removed by inserting a small catheter into the nipple. Saline flows from the catheter into the duct to remove the cells.
    2. Nipple aspiration uses gentle suction to collect fluid from the nipple.

3.   Fine needle aspiration involves inserting a thin needle into the breast tissue to obtain fluid.

Mammotome (Fine, et al., 2003)

- Is a directional, vacuum-assisted, hand-held biopsy device
- Is used for percutaneous removal of palpable and nonpalpable breast masses
- Less time-consuming, nonsurgical procedure done under local anesthesia
- Does not cause disfigurement
- Safe to perform in women with breast implants

Ultrasound (Machia, 2004; Mautner, et al., 2000)

- Also called breast sonography
- Ineffective as a screening method
- Role is to evaluate specific areas of concern raised by mammography and CBE
- Uses
  1. Differentiate between cystic and solid palpable mass
  2. Evaluation of nonpalpable mass
- Benefits
  1. Distinguishes solid from cystic mass
  2. Distinguishes between malignant and nonmalignant mass (e.g., abscess)

- Limitation
  1. Expense

REFERENCES

Blanchard, K., Colbert, J. A., Puri, D., Weissman, J., Moy, B., Kopans, D. B., et al. (2004). Mammographic screening: Patterns of use and estimated impact on breast carcinoma survival. *Cancer, 101*(3), 495–507.

Colbert, J. A., Kaine, E. M., Bigby, J., Smith, D. N., Moore, R. H., Rafferty, E., et al. (2004). The age at which women begin mammographic screening. *Cancer, 101*(8), 1850–1859.

Fabian, C. J., Kimler, B. F., Zalles, C. M., Klemp, J. R., Kamel, S., Zeiger, S., et al. (2000). Short-term breast cancer prediction by random periareolar fine-needle aspiration cytology and the Gail risk model. *Journal of the National Cancer Institute, 92*(15), 1217–1227.

Fine, R. E., Whitworth, P. W., Kim, J. A., Harness, J. K., Boyd, B. A., & Burak, W. E., Jr. (2003). Low-risk palpable breast masses removed using a vacuum-assisted hand-held device. *American Journal of Surgery, 186*(4), 362–367.

Hendrick, R., Smith, R., Rutledge, J., & Smart, C. R. (1997). Benefit of screening mammography in women aged 40–49: A new meta-analysis of randomized controlled trials. *Journal of the National Cancer Institute Monograph, 22*, 87–92.

Machia, J. (2004). Screening and early detection. In K. H. Dow (Ed.), *Contemporary issues in breast cancer: A nursing persective* (2nd ed., pp. 45–57). Sudbury, MA: Jones & Bartlett.

Mautner, B. D., Schmidt, K. V., & Brennan, M. B. (2000). New diagnostic techniques and treatments for early breast cancer. *Seminars in Oncology Nursing, 16*(3), 185–196.

National Cancer Institute. (1997). *Statement from the National Cancer Institute on the National Cancer Advisory Board recommendation on mammography*. Bethesda, MD: National Cancer Institute.

National Cancer Institute. (2004). *NCI Statement on Mammography Screening*. Retrieved October 19, 2004, from www.nci.nih.gov/newscenter/mammstatement31jan02

Sharma, P., Klemp, J. R., Simonsen, M., Welsko, C. M., Zalles, C. M., Kimler, B. F., et al. (2004). Failure of high risk women to produce nipple aspirate fluid does not exclude detection of cytologic atypia in random periareolar fine needle aspiration specimens. *Breast Cancer Research and Treatment, 87*(1), 59–64.

Smith, R., & D'Orsi, C. (2004). Screening for breast cancer. In J. R. Harris, M. Lippman, M. Morrow & C. K. Osborne (Eds.), *Diseases of the breast* (3rd ed., pp. 103–130). Philadelphia: Lippincott Williams & Wilkins.

Smith, R., von Eschenbach, A., Wender, R., & et al. (2001). American Cancer Society guidelines for the early detection of cancer. *CA: A Cancer Journal for Clinicians, 51*, 38–75.

U.K. Trial of Early Detection of Breast Cancer Group. (1999). 16-year mortality from breast cancer in the U.K. trial of early detection of breast cancer. *Lancet, 353*(9168), 1909–1914.

U.S. Preventive Services Task Force. Retrieved October 21, 2004, from www.ahrq.gov/clinic/3rduspstf/breastcancer

CHAPTER FIVE

Diagnosis and Staging

Role of Clinical Breast Examination in Diagnosis
(Foster, 2000)

- Skin may show thickening, redness, dimpling, and/or inflammation.

- Changes in breast shape and variation in normal convexity may indicate an abnormality.

- Changes in appearance of nipple

  Retracted nipple looks flattened or pulled inward.

  Deviation of nipple shows change in the direction in which the nipple normally points.

  Thickening and loss of elasticity of the nipple may be a suspicious finding.

  Persistent scaly or eczema-like lesion may be an indication of Paget's disease.

- Characteristics of malignant breast nodule

  Usually a single nodule

Irregular or stellate shape
Firm or hard consistency
Fixed to skin or underlying tissues
Usually nontender
Retraction may be present

Diagnostic Mammography (Fraker, 2004)

- Diagnostic mammography can detect nonpalpable tumors.
- Mammography can detect about 90% of tumors.
- Detection is more accurate in postmenopausal women because of less tissue density.
- Digital mammography is increasingly used in detection but is more expensive than standard film-screen mammography.
- Mammographic abnormalities include presence of mass and calcifications. Calcifications indicate changes in ducts where breast cancers leave calcium deposits.
- Bilateral mammography is done before biopsy and is indicated for:
  Number and size of the suspicious mass
  Number of masses
  Baseline status
- Mammographic detection more sensitive in postmenopausal women.

Other Diagnostic Imaging Techniques

- Ultrasound or sonography using high-frequency sound waves through the breast

  1. Benefits and uses of ultrasound

     Helps differentiate between cystic and solid lesions

     Helps evaluate lesions in women with dense breast tissue

     Helps distinguish between benign and malignant nonpalpable lesions

  2. Magnetic Resonance Imaging (MRI)

     Can detect small tumors less than 1 cm in size and is useful in imaging dense breasts

     Cost is a major disadvantage

Percutaneous Biopsy of Palpable Lesions

- Techniques depend on the size and characteristics of the mass.

- Types of biopsies for palpable lesions:

  1. Fine-needle aspiration biopsy (FNAB) procedure (Foster, 2000)

     Skin is cleaned with an antiseptic.

     If lesion is solid, a 22-gauge needle may be used with a 20-cc syringe.

     Needle is passed in and out of the lesion several times in various directions.

> *Slight rotary motion allows the bevel of the needle to cut additional cells from the mass.*
>
> *Appearance of aspirated material in the hub shows that an adequate amount of material is aspirated.*
>
> *Suction on the plunger is released, and the needle and syringe are withdrawn.*
>
> *Needle is disconnected from the syringe, and the syringe is filled with air.*
>
> *Needle is replaced and a drop of material is placed onto a glass microscopic slide and spread with another slide.*
>
> *Slides are wet fixed or air dried.*
>
> *Less invasive procedure.*

2. Core-needle biopsy

> *Differs from FNAB in that histologic material is obtained.*
>
> *Core-cutting needle biopsies are processed for permanent or frozen sections.*
>
> *Core-needle biopsies use a spring-loaded, core-cutting needle device, because these devices have decreased pain associated with the biopsy, better diagnostic sensitivity, and provide better specimen quality.*
>
> *Advantages of core-cutting needle biopsy include:*

- Better than excisional or incisional biopsy because it does not require open biopsy.

- False-positive and false-negative rates are low.
- Possibility of seeding the needle track with tumor cells is low.

Percutaneous Biopsy of Nonpalpable Lesions

- Types of biopsies for nonpalpable lesions:
  1. Stereotactic needle-core biopsy

     Stereotactic biopsy is used for lesions detected by a mammogram.

     Two angled radiographic views acquired with the X-ray beam at 15 degrees on either side of the center are used to determine the location of the lesion.

     Computer algorithm uses geometric relations to calculate the position of the lesion based on the shift between the two acquired views.

     Types of stereotactic biopsy units

     1. Dedicated "prone" tables
     2. "Add-on" adapted upright units

  2. Ultrasound-guided needle-core biopsy

     This method is used for masses visualized by an ultrasound.

     Advantage

     1. Preferred by patients because there is no breast compression or radiation

Disadvantage

1. Difficulty in visualizing lesions such as small masses less than 6 mm, calcifications, or architectural distortions

3. Mammotome biopsy

   This method uses a vacuum-assisted system under local anesthesia.

Biopsy of Palpable Lesions

- Excisional biopsy: The surgical removal of entire mass is usually done on an outpatient basis.

  Goal is the removal of the entire mass and surrounding margin of normal tissue.

  It is the definitive treatment for benign lesions.

  For malignant lesions, when a margin of surrounding normal tissue is removed and if pathologic examination confirms that the margins are clean of tumor, then no further breast surgery is needed.

- Incisional biopsy: This is the removal of a portion of a breast mass for pathological evaluation.

  Incisional biopsy is done for diagnostic purposes.

Diagnosis of Breast Cancer

- In-situ carcinomas

  NOS (not otherwise specified)

  Intraductal

  Paget's disease

- Invasive carcinomas

  Infiltrating ductal carcinoma accounts for 75% of invasive breast cancers and presents palpable mass or mammographic abnormalities.

  Infiltrating lobular carcinoma accounts for 5% to 10% of invasive breast cancers.

  Medullary carcinoma accounts for 5% to 7% of invasive breast cancers.

  Mucinous and tubular carcinoma together account for about 5% of invasive breast cancers.

- Inflammatory

  This accounts for less than 5% of invasive breast cancer.

Staging of Breast Cancer

- The staging of breast cancer is determined by the American Joint Committee on Cancer (AJCC).
- The AJCC system is a clinical and pathologic staging system based on the TNM classification (tumor, nodes, metastasis) (see Table 5-1).
- Clinical staging is based on physical examination.
- Pathologic staging is based on data used for clinical staging, surgical resection, and pathologic examination of the primary carcinoma.
- Primary *tumor* is the size of the breast lesion.
- *Nodes* refers to the involvement of regional lymph nodes.

TABLE 5-1
Classification and Staging of Breast Cancer

Stage	Tumor (T)	Nodes (N)	Metastasis (M)
		Characteristics	
Stage 0	Carcinoma in situ	No regional lymph node metastasis	No distant metastasis
Stage I	Tumor of 2 cm or less	No axillary node involvement	No distant metastasis
Stage IIA			
T0 N1 M0	No tumor	Movable ipsilateral axillary node involvement	No distant metastasis
T1 N1 M0	Tumor 2 cm or less	Movable ipsilateral axillary node involvement	No distant metastasis
T2 N0 M0	Tumor 2–5 cm	No nodal involvement	No distant metastasis
Stage IIB			
T2 N1 M0	Tumor 2–5 cm	Movable ipsilateral axillary node involvement	No distant metastasis
T3 N0 M0	Tumor >5 cm	No nodal involvement	No distant metastasis
Stage IIIA			
T0 N2 M0	No tumor	Ipsilateral axillary lymph node(s) fixed to one another or to other structures	No distant metastasis

(continues)

TABLE 5-1 (*continued*)
Classification and Staging of Breast Cancer

Stage	Tumor (T)	Nodes (N)	Metastasis (M)
		Characteristics	
T1 N2 M0	Tumor <2 cm	Ipsilateral axillary nodes containing tumor growth and fixed to one another or other structures	No distant metastasis
T2 N2 M0	Tumor >2 cm but <5 cm	Ipsilateral axillary lymph nodes fixed to one another or to other structures	No distant metastasis
T3 N1 M0	Tumor >5 cm	Movable ipsilateral axillary node involvement	No distant metastasis
T3 N2 M0	Tumor >5 cm	Ipsilateral axillary lymph nodes fixed to one another or to other structures	No metastasis
Stage IIIB			
T4 N0 M0	Tumor of any size with direct extension to chest wall	No regional lymph node metastasis	No distant metastasis
T4 N1 M0	Tumor of any size with direct extension to chest wall	Metastasis to movable ipsilateral axillary lymph node	No distant metastasis

(continues)

TABLE 5-1 (*continued*)
Classification and Staging of Breast Cancer

Stage	Tumor (T)	Nodes (N)	Metastasis (M)
		Characteristics	
T4 N2 M0	Tumor of any size with direct extension to chest wall	Metastasis in ipsilateral axillary lymph nodes fixed or matted	No distant metastasis
Stage IIIC Any T N3 M0	Tumor of any size with direct extension to chest wall	Metastasis in ipsilateral infraclavicular lymph nodes with or without axillary lymph node involvement	No distant metastasis
Stage IV Any T Any N M1	Tumor of any size with direct extension to chest wall or skin	Any N	Distant metastasis

Source: Used with the permission of the American Joint Committee on Cancer (AJCC), Chicago, Illinois. The original source for this material is the AJCC Cancer Staging Manual, Sixth Edition (2002) published by Springer-Verlag New York, www.springeronline.com

Level I nodes (low axilla): Lymph nodes lateral to the lateral border of the pectoralis minor muscle

Level II nodes (mid-axilla): Lymph nodes between the medial and lateral borders of the pectoralis minor muscle and the interpectoral (Rotter's) lymph nodes

Level III (apical axilla): Lymph nodes medial to the medial margin of the pectoralis minor muscle, including those designated as subclavicular, infravicular, or apical

Internal mammary (ipsilateral): Lymph nodes in the intercostal spaces along the edge of the sternum in the endothoracic fascia

Other lymph nodes, including the supraclavicular, cervical, or contralateral internal mammary nodes, are coded as distant metastasis.

- Additional Staging Procedures

In general, patients with early stage disease have a physical examination and blood chemistry done before surgery.

Decisions about additional procedures are often recommended after surgery.

1. If alkaline phosphatase levels are elevated, a bone scan can be considered to evaluate presence of bone metastasis.

2. Chest radiograph can be used to evaluate asymptomatic pulmonary metastasis.

3. Liver scan, liver ultrasound, or computed tomography scan of liver may be recommended if liver function tests are elevated.

Sentinel Lymph Node Mapping and Dissection
(Fraker, 2004)

- The role of sentinel lymph node (SLN) mapping is to ensure adequate staging while minimizing complications, provide for regional control of disease, and have the potential for small therapeutic benefit.

- The American Society of Breast Surgeons' Consensus Statement on Guidelines for Performance of Sentinel Lymphadenectomy for breast cancer is located at: www.breastsurgeons.org/officialstmts/sentinel.shtml

- Definition: Removal of sentinel lymph node (first draining lymph node from tumor bed).

- When the sentinel lymph node is identified and when lymphatic drainage occurs in an organized pattern of progression, the sentinel lymph node reflects the pathologic status of the nodes.

- When the sentinel lymph node is biopsied and is pathologically free of cancer cells, then remaining nodes in the axilla are considered negative for cancer.

- Axillary node dissection may not be needed when the sentinel lymph node is negative, thus increasing potential for axillary complications.

- Procedure

    Blue dye is injected around the primary lesion and traced to the first blue node or sentinel node.

Gamma probe mapping, using 99m Technetium-labeled sulfur colloid injected (radionuclide) preoperatively into the breast mass and combined with a trace using a probe that is sensitive to gamma rays. Migration of radionuclide to the axilla is confirmed by lymphoscintigraphy and a gamma ray probe.

In combination with intraoperative lymphatic mapping, the procedure helps to decrease the risk associated with axillary node dissection (such as paresthesias, drains, immobility, cutaneous numbness, limited arm movement, fluid collection, and lymphedema).

Prognostic Markers (Chang & Hilsenbeck, 2004)

- Prognostic markers are factors that characterize the aggressiveness of cancer and are used in staging and determination of treatment

  Nodal status

  Tumor size

  Pathologic subtype

  Nuclear grade

  Steroid receptor status

  Estrogen receptor

  Progesterone receptor

  HER2/neu overexpression

Predictive Markers

- Predictive markers are factors that are used to evaluate an individual's response to treatment.

- Estrogen receptor predicts response to hormonal therapy.

- HER2/neu amplification predicts response to trastuzumab.

REFERENCES

Chang, J., & Hilsenbeck, S. (2004). Prognostic and predictive markers. In J. Harris, M. Lippman, M. Morrow & C. K. Osborne (Eds.), *Diseases of the breast* (3rd ed., pp. 676–696). Philadelphia: Lippincott Williams & Wilkins.

Foster, R. (2000). Techniques of diagnosis of palpable breast masses. In J. Harris, M. Lippman, M. Morrow & C. Osborne (Eds.), *Diseases of the breast* (2nd ed., pp. 95–100). Philadelphia: Lippincott Williams & Wilkins.

Fraker, T. (2004). Diagnosis and staging. In K. H. Dow (Ed.), *Contemporary issues in breast cancer: A nursing perspective* (2nd ed., pp. 58–79). Sudbury, MA: Jones & Bartlett.

Greene, F. L., Page, D. L., Fleming, I. D., et al. (2002). AJCC Cancer Staging Manual, Sixth Edition. New York: Springer-Verlag, 2002.

PART II

Treatment of Primary Breast Cancer

CHAPTER SIX

Surgical Techniques

Use of Surgery in Breast Cancer

- Treatment of noninvasive breast cancer
- Modified radical mastectomy (MRM)
- Total mastectomy
- Breast conservation treatment (BCT)
- Axillary lymph node dissection (ALND) or sampling
- Sentinel lymph node mapping and dissection (SLN)

Noninvasive (In-Situ) Breast Cancer

- Aim of treatment is to prevent occurrence of invasive disease
- Types of noninvasive breast cancer
  Ductal carcinoma in situ (DCIS)
  Lobular carcinoma in situ (LCIS)

- National Comprehensive Cancer Network (NCCN) guidelines for the treatment of DCIS and LCIS can be accessed online at www.nccn.org/professionals/physician_gls/PDF/breast.pdf

Ductal Carcinoma in Situ (DCIS) (Morrow & Harris, 2004)

- DCIS is known as intraductal carcinoma.
- With the widespread use of screening mammography, 16% to 18% of breast cancers diagnosed annually are DCIS.
- Prior to screening mammography, DCIS was an unusual finding.
- Microcalcifications are the most common mammographic finding in DCIS.
- Linear and heterogeneous morphology is associated with cancer, while random calcifications throughout the breast are considered benign.
- DCIS is a precursor with a variable risk of progression, depending on histology, lesion, size, and multicentricity.

  There is a 30% risk of invasive cancer with DCIS after 10 years

  DCIS is associated with an excellent prognosis.

- Treatment of DCIS as primary diagnosis

  Mastectomy is curative in 98% of patients and has been recommended in patients with extensive DCIS and microcalcifications.

Excision and radiation therapy reduces risk of recurrence compared with excision alone in low-risk patients.

Excision and tamoxifen recommended in low-risk patients with ER+ DCIS.

Excision alone is being evaluated in older patients with small, low-grade DCIS.

Lobular Neoplasia: Lobular Carcinoma In-Situ (LCIS)

- LCIS is considered a risk factor or marker of abnormal proliferative activity rather than a pre-cursor to breast cancer.

- Chemoprevention with tamoxifen reduces the risk of breast cancer in women with LCIS (Fisher, et al., 1998).

- LCIS is not detected on a mammogram and is usu-ally diagnosed by biopsy of a lesion.

- LCIS is associated with an increased risk of invasive breast cancer.

- LCIS was first described in 1941 as a noninvasive form of breast cancer that arises in the lobules and terminal ducts.

- Lesion is usually an asymptomatic, incidental micro-scopic finding that does not show as a mass on mammography.

- It is considered a risk factor or marker of abnormal proliferative activity rather than a precursor to breast cancer.

LCIS is seen more often in younger women.

*LCIS is usually found on biopsy as a histologic compo-
nent in pathologic specimens after surgery.*

- Current treatment for primary LCIS ranges from
  observation, risk reduction to bilateral mastectomy.
- Chemoprevention with tamoxifen reduces risk of
  breast cancer in women with LCIS.

Modified Radical Mastectomy

- MRM is the most common surgical treatment for
  breast cancer in the United States.
- Mastectomy as a primary treatment reduces tumor
  mass and increases the effectiveness of systemic
  therapy.
- Procedure:

  *Removal of the entire breast: nipple/areolar complex and
  pectoral fascia*

  Level I, II, or III axillary lymph node dissection

  Pectoralis major is preserved

- Indications for mastectomy

  Large, bulky tumors

  Multicentric disease

  *Likelihood that the cosmetic outcome of breast-conserving
  surgery and radiation therapy may be poor*

  Patient preference and choice

- NCCN Guidelines for the locoregional treatment of invasive breast cancer with mastectomy can be accessed online at www.nccn.org/professionals/ physician_gls/PDF/breast.pdf

Total Mastectomy

- Involves removal of the entire breast, with preservation of the pectoral muscles and axillary nodes
- Candidates for total mastectomy
    1. Patients with DCIS
    2. Patients undergoing prophylactic mastectomy
    3. Patients who develop recurrence in the breast after breast-conserving surgery and radiation therapy

Complications of Mastectomy (Morrow & Harris, 2000)

- Wound infection

    Cellulitis occurs in early postoperative period.

    Abscess formation may occur as a late effect.

- Risk factors for infection

    Use of a two-step procedure with open biopsy and mastectomy.

    Prolonged suction catheter drainage.

- Necrosis of skin flaps is uncommon.
- Factors associated with necrosis of skin flaps:

Denuding subcutaneous fat from flap

Closure of wound under tension

Infection

Occlusive pressure dressings

Vertical incisions (currently not used)

- Phantom breast sensation

    About 50% of patients experience a residual sensation of the breast after mastectomy.

    Symptoms include pain, itching, nipple sensation, erotic sensation, and premenstrual-type soreness.

    Cause of phantom breast sensation is unknown, and symptoms may be constant over time.

Breast-Conserving Surgery

- BCT involves removal, wide excision of tumor and margin of normal surrounding tissue with preservation of the breast.
- BCT and radiation therapy (XRT) is considered the standard treatment for most women with stage I and II breast cancer.
- Incidence of recurrence with BCT is 3% to 19%.
- BCT failure is treated with mastectomy.
- No survival difference with BCT + XRT compared with mastectomy.
- Reader is referred to Chapter 8 for further information about treatment with XRT for primary breast cancer.

Axillary Lymph Node Dissection

- The number of involved axillary lymph nodes at the diagnosis is one of the most important prognostic indicators in breast cancer.

- Axillary lymph nodes are the major regional drainage site for the breast, receiving 85% of lymphatic drainage.

- Likelihood that axillary nodes are involved with tumor is related to the size of the primary tumor, histologic grade, and presence of lymphatic invasion.

- Axillary nodes are divided into three levels based on their anatomic relationship to the pectoralis minor muscle.

- ALND is responsible for the major morbidity associated with breast cancer, including lymphedema, injury or thrombosis of the axillary vein, and injury to motor nerves in the axilla.

- Other morbidity associated with ALND includes seroma formation, shoulder dysfunction, and loss of sensation in the distribution of the intercostobrachial nerve.

- There is increased attention as to the value of ALND in women with early-stage primary breast cancer.

- ALND may be considered an option in selected patients:

  Patients with favorable tumors

  Elderly patients

Patients with serious concurrent morbidity

Patients for whom selection of adjuvant therapy or hormonal therapy is not likely to be affected by evaluation of nodal status

- Patient information on lymphedema management after axillary node dissection is contained in Figure 6-1.

Sentinel Lymph Node Biopsy

- Sentinel node is the first node that drains lymph from a cancer (Giuliano, et al., 1997; Hsueh, 2000; Pendas, et al., 2004).

- If the sentinel lymph node is negative for the presence of malignancy, the rest of the axillary lymph nodes may be negative for disease.

- Table 6-1 outlines the advantages and limitations of sentinel lymph node biopsy compared with axillary node dissection.

- Contraindications to SLNB include:

Palpable lymph node adenopathy

Tumors larger than 5 cm in size or locally advanced breast cancer

Use of preoperative chemotherapy

Multifocal disease

Prior major breast or axillary surgery that may interfere with lymphatic drainage

Pregnant or lactating patient

FIGURE 6–1

Patient Information on Lymphedema Management After Axillary Node Dissection

The lymph nodes that are located in the axilla will be removed to determine whether the nodes have any cancer cells. Lymph nodes are located throughout the body. They filter fluids, proteins and bacteria that are in our bodies. Occasionally, after the lymph nodes have been removed, it causes an ineffective filtering of this fluid, which sometimes results in edema (fluid accumulation) in the arm. The following guidelines have been established to prevent lymphedema from occurring. It is important to review these guidelines and incorporate them into your daily lifestyle.

1. Good skin hygiene; use lotion after bathing. When drying the arm, be gentle, but thorough.

2. Avoid venipuncture, injections and infusions in the affected arm.

3. Wear protective gloves when working outside or with cleaning products.

4. Wear sunscreen to protect against sunburn and use insect repellent to protect against bites and stings.

5. Do not cut hangnails or cut nails too short; do not push cuticles back to the nailbed.

6. Exercise and use the affected arm. Full range of motion and strength of affected arm should return in a couple of months.

You can expect to resume all your activities of daily living, i.e., swimming, golfing, tennis, without any compromise to the affected arm within a few months.

If you should experience a cut, scrape or burn to the affected arm, clean the area thoroughly, use an antiseptic and cover the area with a bandage. If you should notice any redness, swelling, or tenderness contact your physician immediately. You may need to take an antibiotic.

TABLE 6-1
Advantages and Limitations of Sentinel Lymph Node Biopsy

Advantages of SLNB over ALND	Limitations of SLNB
Less invasive than level I–II axillary dissection	Possible false-negative results
May be more sensitive to detecting lymph node metastases	Not suitable for all patients (age and location of tumor limit success rate)
Potential to eliminate routine ALND for patients whose sentinel node is negative	Needs further technical improvements and studies

Preoperative Patient Education (Lynn, 2004)

- Reinforce information and treatment recommendations.

- Answer questions about hospital procedures, surgical experience, and follow-up home management.

- Provide teaching materials, pamphlets, booklets, and Web sites dedicated to information about breast cancer and surgery.

- Assess baseline circumference of both arms prior to surgery.

- Measure 5 and 10 cm above and below the olecranon process.

- Changes in preoperative baseline can be compared with postoperative measurement.

- Instruct the patient to avoid aspirin and aspirin-containing products and vitamin E supplements at least 7 days prior to surgery.

- Instruct the patient to discuss herbal preparations with anesthesiologist.
- Referral to "Reach for Recovery" prior to mastectomy.

Postmastectomy Nursing Care

- Because patients have a short length of inpatient stay, nursing care will concentrate on immediate postoperative care and teaching the patient self-care after discharge.
- Major areas of focus for immediate postoperative care include:

  Managing pain

  Monitoring for hematoma, flap necrosis, and infection on day of surgery

  Assessing the patient's psychosocial response

- Major areas of focus for self-care after discharge include:

  Help the patient view the incisional site.

  Teach the patient about incision care.

  Examine the site for healing and prevention of infection.

  Demonstrate how to empty and measure serous fluid from the drain, if present after discharge (Figure 6-2 lists drain care after surgery).

  Demonstrate how to strip tubing and remove clots.

  Provide a teaching pamphlet/booklet on exercises.

  Discuss the importance of arm and hand exercises.

  Discuss exercises to maintain range of motion.

  Improve collateral circulation.

FIGURE 6-2
Patient Information Sheet for Drain Care After Surgery

After surgery, you will have a bulb like reservoir connected to tubing coming from your incision. This device suctions and collects fluid from your incision area. The drain promotes healing and reduces the chance of infection. This drain will be in place for several days after surgery. When you go home with the drain, here is how you should care for it:

1. Empty the drain every 8 to 12 hours. You will be provided with a small cup with measurement markings on the side. Empty the drain into the cup so that you can accurately record how much drainage you have.

2. Unpin the drainage bulb from your bra or shirt.

   Remove the rubber stopper from the drain. Turn the drain upside down, and squeeze the contents into the measuring cup. Completely empty the bulb.

   Keep a record of the amount of fluid in the measuring cup.

   Note: To prevent infection, don't let the rubber stopper or top of the drain touch the measuring cup or any other surface.

3. Now, use one hand to squeeze all of the air from the drain. With the drain still compressed, use your other hand to replace the rubber stopper. Do this to ensure the drain suction works well.

Postdischarge Patient Self-Care

- Patients must learn how to change the surgical dressing.

  Manage surgical drains.

  Monitor for signs of infection.

  Continue hand and arm exercises 20 minutes a day, three times a week.

- Maintain adequate nutritional and fluid intake to help healing of the incision.
- Adapt home management techniques.

  Rest and relaxation

  Stress management

  Permit others to help with home, family, or work responsibilities
- Manage postoperative pain.

  Take prescribed medication.

  Assess for arm sensations (after axillary dissection).

  Assess for numbness, tingling, burning in axilla.

  Presence of arm sensations is normal.

Postdischarge Nursing Care Issues

- Review plans for the next step in cancer treatment and referral to radiation therapy and chemotherapy and hormonal therapy.
- Review plans for surgical follow-up.
- Assess the patient's psychosocial response.
- Discuss whether the patient may be interested in accessing individual or support groups.
- Suggest community resources for assistance.
- Reinforce teaching and support for

  Postmastectomy exercises

  Lymphedema prevention

  Management of fatigue

Help with body-image changes
Referral to prosthetist when necessary

REFERENCES

Fisher, B., Costantino, J., Wickerham, D., & et al. (1998). Tamoxifen for prevention of breast cancer: Report of the National Surgical Adjuvant Breast and Bowel Project P-1 Study. *Journal of the National Cancer Institute, 16,* 1381–1388.

Giuliano, A. E., Jones, R. C., Brennan, M., & et al. (1997). Sentinel lymphadenectomy in breast cancer. *Journal of Clinical Oncology, 15,* 2345–2350.

Hsueh, E. C., Hansen, H., & Giuliano, A. E. (2000). Intraoperative lymphatic mapping and sentinel lymph node dissection in breast cancer. *CA: A Cancer Journal for Clinicians, 50,* 279–291.

Lynn, J. (2004). Surgery techniques. In K. H. Dow (Ed.), *Contemporary issues in breast cancer: A nursing persective* (2nd ed., pp. 81–89). Sudbury, MA: Jones & Bartlett.

Morrow, M., & Harris, J. (2004). Ductal carcinoma in situ and microinvasive carcinoma. In J. R. Harris, M. E. Lippman, M. Morrow & C. K. Osborne (Eds.), *Diseases of the breast* (3rd ed., pp. 521–537). Philadelphia: Lippincott Williams & Wilkins.

Morrow, M., & Harris, J. R. (2000). Primary treatment of invasive breast cancer. In J. R. Harris, M. Lippman, M. Morrow, & C. K. Osborne (Eds.), *Diseases of the breast* (2nd ed., pp. 515–560). Philadelphia: Lippincott Williams & Wilkins.

Pendas, S., Giuliano, R., Swor, G., Gardner, M., Jakub, J., & Reintgen, D. S. (2004). Worldwide experience with lymphatic mapping for invasive breast cancer. *Seminars in Oncology, 31*(3), 318–323.

CHAPTER SEVEN

Reconstructive Surgery

Breast Reconstruction (Baron & Vaziri, 2004; Fine & Mustoe, 2004)

- Elective surgery to enhance self-image after mastectomy
- Goal: To alleviate the deformity in the chest wall and breast after mastectomy
- Considered an important part of cancer rehabilitation
- Rationale for choosing breast reconstruction

    Helps restore body symmetry

    Helps decrease feelings of loss and disfigurement

    Helps restore sense of femininity and sexuality

    Helps to decrease reminder of breast cancer as a life-threatening illness

    Improves ability to wear clothing

> *Decreases feelings of embarrassment about the prosthesis*
>
> *Helps improve body image*

- Reasons why women do not have breast reconstruction

  Older age

  Concern about a second surgical procedure

  Uncertainty over the cosmetic outcome

  Fear of discomfort and pain

  Additional cost and expense

- What is the best breast reconstruction?

  No single best procedure for all women

  Decision about breast reconstruction and type is an individual one, based on risks and benefits

- Timing of breast reconstruction

  Immediate or delayed reconstruction based on patient preference and choice

  Immediate reconstruction performed in a majority of procedures today

  No differences noted in survival or recurrence rates with immediate or delayed reconstruction

Immediate Reconstruction

- It is a safe procedure that does not delay adjuvant therapy.
- One surgical procedure is a cost-effective treatment.

- It may help with body image adjustment and provide greater psychological benefit, compared with delayed reconstruction.
- Federal laws in the United States require insurance companies to cover breast reconstruction after mastectomy.

Delayed Reconstruction

- Gives the patient time to adjust after the initial mastectomy procedure
- Provides the patient with additional time to make an informed decision
- May be done up to several days to years after mastectomy
- Requires a second surgical procedure
- May result in a more visible scarring of the reconstructed breast
- Need for postoperative radiation may require delayed reconstruction
- Table 7-1 outlines the technical consideration in using immediate or delayed reconstruction.

Types of Breast Reconstruction

- Expander/implant
- Autologous reconstruction
- Table 7-2 compares the various reconstructive procedures (Baron & Vaziri, 2004).

TABLE 7-1

Technical Considerations in Immediate and Delayed
Reconstruction

Immediate Reconstruction	*Delayed Reconstruction*
Less scar formation with stiffening and contracture occurs.	Mastopexy may be needed to achieve breast symmetry.
Breast is more malleable.	Tissue expander with delayed reconstruction allows skin to heal and decreases risk of mastectomy flap breakdown.
Concurrent flap harvest during mastectomy, assisted elevation of mastectomy skin flaps help expedite procedure.	Elevation of contracted, fibrotic skin flaps requires larger inset from the abdomen, leading to a less natural result.
Preservation of inframammary fold and use of skin-sparing mastectomies help lead to a natural and symmetric reconstruction.	

Expander/Implant (Fine & Mustoe, 2004)

- Tissue expansion, followed by removal of the expander and placement of the permanent implant.

- Most common form of breast reconstruction in the United States.

- Procedure is recommended for women with small- to moderate-sized contralateral breasts with little ptosis and healthy flaps.

TABLE 7-2
Comparison of Reconstruction Procedures

Surgical procedure	Anesthesia	OR time	Days in hospital	Shape and consistency	Scars
Tissue expander	General	1 hr	2–3 with mastectomy, ambulatory if delayed	No natural ptosis, firm	No new scars
Latissimus dorsi flap	General	3–4 hrs	2–4	Natural shape, soft	Donor-site scar on back
Pedicle TRAM flap	General	4–5 hrs	4–5	Natural shape, soft	Donor-site scar on abdomen
Free TRAM flap	General	5–6 hrs	5–7	Natural shape, soft	Donor-site scar on abdomen
Gluteal free flap	General	6–8 hrs	7–10	Natural shape, soft	Donor-site scar on gluteus

Procedures done following initial breast reconstruction:

. Nipple/ areolar reconstruction: ambulatory surgery done under local anesthesia with IV sedation; procedure time 1.5 hrs.

Exchange from temporary tissue expander to permanent breast implant: ambulatory surgery done under general anesthesia; procedure time 1 hour.

- Technical improvements in saline expanders and implants that are contoured and textured have improved the overall cosmetic outcome.

- Implants do not match the natural shape and curve of the natural breast.

- Tissue expansion/permanent implant

  Tissue expansion is the process by which the skin and pectoralis muscle are stretched after mastectomy in order to accommodate a permanent implant.

  Tissue expander is a balloon-like device inserted under the pectoralis muscle either at the time of mastectomy or at the time of delayed reconstruction.

  Small amount of saline is inserted into a port in the expander to partially inflate the expander.

  About 2 weeks after mastectomy, the tissue is expanded by inserting additional saline into the expander. Process is repeated weekly for about 6–8 weeks.

  Permanent implant is exchanged for the tissue expander about 3 months after surgery.

  Complications of tissue expansion/permanent implant

    1. Capsular contracture; treated with open capsulotomy (cutting of the scar tissue) or capsulectomy (removal of scar tissue)

    2. Infection

    3. Mastectomy flap necrosis

    4. Implant rupture or deflation

- Complications of the expander/implant are less than 10% in women who do not have postoperative radiation.

- Choice of a saline versus a silicone gel implant for breast reconstruction depends on preference and choice (see Table 7-3).

  Reconstructive techniques have changed within the past 10 years. When silicone implants were placed in a single-stage procedure without tissue expansion, there was a higher risk of complications.

  In patients with postoperative radiation, the complication rate may increase up to 18%.

- Contraindications to expander/implant

  Absolute contraindication is infection or lack of viable skin flap to close over the expander.

TABLE 7-3

Comparison Between Saline and Silicone Gel Implants

Saline Implant	Silicone Gel Implant
Predominant choice over silicone gel	Available on investigational basis only
Firm and holds shape	Concern over link with connective tissue disorders, although studies do not demonstrate a relationship
Less likely to develop contracture	Softer and more natural feeling and texture
Contracture with silicone gel makes for a harder implant	Implant leakage and silicone gel bleed may occur over time

> *Relative contraindications include prior radiation,*
> *planned postoperative radiation, obesity, and*
> *smoking history.*

Autologous Reconstruction

- Transverse rectus abdominus myocutaneous (TRAM) flap
- Latissimus dorsi myocutaneous flap

Transverse Rectus Abdominis Myocutaneous Flap

- TRAM is the most widely used autologous procedure.
- The procedure uses skin and fatty tissue from the lower abdomen to replace the skin (nipple and biopsy site) and breast tissue removed during mastectomy.
- The rectus abdominis muscle is used as a conduit for blood flow to overlying subcutaneous fat and skin of the lower abdomen.
- The TRAM flap replaces tissue lost with autologous tissue, which achieves a natural look and feel that is not possible with expander/implants.
- The patient must have adequate abdominal tissue, be a nonsmoker, and be in good physical condition to undergo long recovery.
- The procedure can be initiated concurrently with mastectomy to reduce operative time.
- Complications: partial flap loss, delayed healing

- Absolute contraindications to TRAM flap are prior upper abdominal incision with division of rectus abdominis and abdominoplasty.

- Relative contraindications are older age, poor health, history of smoking, obesity, diabetes, hypertension, and thinness (e.g., not having enough lower abdominal tissue available for the procedure).

Free TRAM Flap

- This is a modification of the conventional TRAM flap to minimize problems of secondary blood supply and the need for extensive dissection.

- A portion of rectus muscle, fat, and skin is detached from abdominal site and blood supply. Tissue is transplanted to the mastectomy site.

- Patients who may benefit from free TRAM include smokers, the obese, and other high-risk patients, and patients requiring bilateral reconstruction.

- The procedure has the advantages of a reliable primary blood supply, limits dissection, and provides improved recovery after surgery.

- Free TRAM is based on the deep inferior epigastric vessels, which are the primary blood supply to the lower abdomen.

- The procedure is complex using microsurgery.

- Complications: total flap loss, partial flap loss, fat necrosis, bleeding and thrombosis.

Latissimus Dorsi Musculocutaneous Flap

- Procedure involves the rotation of the lattisimus muscle with ellipse of skin from the mastectomy site.

- It is less commonly used in comparison to the TRAM flap, but high patient satisfaction and a low number of complications have increased the popularity of this procedure.

- It serves as an alternative to TRAM for women with inadequate skin at the mastectomy site, abdominal scarring, or prior abdominal surgical procedures.

- Patients who have had prior radiation therapy have lower capsular contraction because the implants are covered by nonirradiated tissue.

- Patients who require postoperative radiation after immediate reconstruction with the latissimus flap have a higher incidence of capsular contraction.

- If a large amount of skin is removed, this procedure provides an excellent cosmetic result.

- Drawbacks: Skin color and texture may differ from that of the breast.

- Long-term results show that latissimus dorsi reconstruction is associated with high patient satisfaction, moderate capsular contracture rates, and minor flap loss.

- Complications: prolonged seroma, capsular contraction, and infection.

Bilateral Free TRAM Flap

- Bilateral autologous reconstruction.
- It is used for women having contralateral or prophylactic mastectomy.
- Women who have sequential mastectomies are not candidates for the TRAM flap.
- Bilateral pedicled TRAM breast reconstruction:

  Requires sufficient lower abdominal tissue

  Takes about 6 to 8 hours

  Has prolonged recovery

  Associated with an increase in abdominal weakness

- In comparison, bilateral free TRAM flap reconstruction may be beneficial for patients with active lifestyles and for high-risk patients.

  Flaps can be harvested at the same time the mastectomy is performed.

  Blood supply decreases fat necrosis and allows for better breast contouring.

  Vascularity of the upper abdominal skin flap is preserved because extensive tunneling is not needed.

  Benefits include good cosmetic outcome and lower abdominal morbidity.

Nipple–Areolar Reconstruction

- Nipple reconstruction helps to enhance final cosmetic outcome.

- Nipple reconstruction allows for a more natural-appearing "breast."

- Generally done after completion of reconstruction as a second-stage procedure in conjunction with mound revision or a contralateral symmetry procedure (e.g., breast reduction, mastopexy, or augmentation).

- Procedure may be done after completing adjuvant therapy.

- Micropigmentation or areolar tattooing achieves a natural color.

- When needed, full-thickness skin grafts may be harvested from the groin or excess skin from the TRAM flap.

Nursing Management (Baron & Vaziri, 2004)

- Reconstruction minimizes the negative effects of breast cancer and treatment. Women choose reconstruction through a decision-making process of getting one's life back (Neill, et al., 1998).

- Teaching points

  Reconstructed breast may approximate the look but will not look exactly like the former breast.

  Patient may experience fewer sensations in the reconstructed breast.

- Table 7-4 lists general preoperative topics and teaching points to review with patients.

- Table 7-5 reviews procedure-specific teaching points to review with patients.

TABLE 7-4
General Preoperative Teaching

Topics to Cover Preoperatively	Teaching Points
Things to expect after surgery	Patients undergoing a flap procedure will have an incision and surgical drain(s) at the reconstructed breast site and at the donor site.
	Postoperative swelling is normal and may last for a couple of weeks.
	There may be temporary skin-color changes at the reconstructed site (bruising, pinkish skin). These changes improve with time.
	Patients undergoing a flap procedure will experience temporary tightness at the reconstructed site and at the donor site.
	Any patients having a flap procedure will have a Foley catheter for 2–3 days postoperatively.
	Patients having TRAM or gluteal flap procedure are asked to donate 1–2 units of packed red blood cells in case it is needed during or after surgery.
	Patients are taught breathing and leg exercises to prevent pneumonia and DVT, respectively.

(*continues*)

TABLE 7-4 (*continued*)
General Preoperative Teaching

Topics to Cover Preoperatively	Teaching Points
Change in sensation in the reconstructed breast	Patients may experience temporary changes in sensation such as sensitivity to touch, numbness, and tingling (caused by nerve damage during mastectomy). Some degree of numbness and change of sensation may be permanent.
Pain management	Pain medication may include PCA pumps, IM, or PO narcotics depending on level of pain (e.g., morphine, Percocet, Darvocet).
Range-of-motion exercises	Exercises generally begin the day after surgery with appropriate modifications for individual procedures.
Home-care needs	Patients having TRAM flap or gluteal flap will need help at home for at least 1 week following discharge.
Time away from work	Approximately 4–6 weeks after implant reconstruction 6–8 weeks after latissimus dorsi flap 6–12 weeks after TRAM flap and gluteal flap

TABLE 7-5
Procedure-Specific Teaching Points

Topics to Cover Preoperatively	Teaching Points
Tissue expander/implant reconstruction	Provide patients with clothing hints to maximize symmetry and improve their appearance during expansion process.
	Instruct patients not to have MRI with tissue expander because port is metal.
	Metal in the port may set off alarm at security checkpoints in airport.
	Instruct patients to permanently avoid exercises that will develop the pectoralis muscle, which can result in distortion of the reconstructed breast.
	Instruct patients to pad seat belt when traveling long distances in a car if seat belt falls directly over the implant.
Latissimus dorsi flap reconstruction	Donor-site incision line causes great deal of tension in the back.
	Patients will have difficulty extending arm above head for 2–3 weeks. They should not prematurely force the movement.
	Avoid extreme stretching exercises (advanced yoga) for 6–8 weeks to prevent dehiscence of donor-site incision line.
TRAM-flap reconstruction	Abdominal donor-site incision causes great deal of tension in abdominal area.

(continues)

TABLE 7-5 (*continued*)
Procedure-Specific Teaching Points

Topics to Cover Preoperatively	Teaching Points
	To prevent abdominal spasm or dehiscence of incision line, instruct patients to sleep with head elevated 45 degrees and knees bent or on their side in the fetal position during first postoperative week. In free TRAM flap, range of motion exercises are delayed 7–10 days to prevent tension on anastomosed vessels.
Gluteal free-flap reconstruction	Patients must avoid lying on their back or on their donor side for 4 weeks because of presence of drains and incision line location. Patients must avoid physical activities/movements that could cause tension on posterior thigh until complete healing at donor-site incision.
Nipple/areolar reconstruction	Avoid direct friction on skin-grafted nipple/areola for 2 weeks (i.e., no shoulder strap on affected side). For first two weeks, pad seat-belt strap if it falls directly on reconstructed site. Avoid lower extremity exercises for 3–4 weeks to prevent dehiscence of skin-graft donor site in upper-inner thigh.

Note: Time frames mentioned may vary depending on physician/nurse experience and preference/condition of patient.

- Postsurgical breast reconstruction nursing care

  Prevention of infection

  Pain management

  Flap assessment: color, temperature, edema

  Management of surgical wound

  Prevention of seroma formation

  Emotional support and body-image assessment

- Table 7-6 identifies areas of assessment of flap condition after Free TRAM flap or Gluteal Free Flap.

TABLE 7-6

Assessment of Flap Condition After Microvascular Surgery (Free TRAM Flap or Gluteal Free Flap)

Assessment Categories	What to Look for
Color	Pink: good color
	Pallor: decreased arterial blood flow
	Mottling: venous congestion
Circulation with Doppler study	Decreased or absent blood flow indicates blockage of anastomosed vessels
Capillary refill	Press on flap to check refill
	Normal refill 3 seconds
	Arterial problem if >5 seconds
	Venous problem if <2 seconds
Temperature	Flap temperature should not be <30 degrees centigrade

Frequency of flap checks: every hour for first 2 days; every 2 hours for second 2 days; every 4 hours for last 2 days.

REFERENCES

Baron, R., & Vaziri, N. (2004). Reconstructive surgery. In K. H. Dow (Ed.), *Contemporary issues in breast cancer* (2nd ed., pp. 105–106). Sudbury, MA: Jones & Bartlett.

Fine, N. A., & Mustoe, T. A. (2004). Breast reconstruction. In J. R. Harris, M. Lippman, M. Morrow, & C. K. Osborne (Eds.), *Diseases of the breast* (3rd ed., pp. 802–818). Philadelphia: Lippincott Williams & Wilkins.

Neill, K., Armstrong, N., & Burnett, C. (1998). Choosing reconstruction after mastectomy: A qualitative analysis. *Oncology Nursing Forum, 25,* 743–750.

CHAPTER EIGHT

Radiation Therapy

Background (Morrow & Harris, 2004; Perun, 2004)

- In the 1900s, radiation therapy (XRT) was first used to treat patients with chest wall recurrence after surgery and as the primary treatment for patients with advanced breast cancer.

- Its role in the local management of breast cancer has changed significantly over the past hundred years.

Uses of Radiation Therapy in Breast Cancer

- Primary local treatment in combination with breast-conserving surgery (BCS)

- Postmastectomy XRT (Wong & Harris, 2004)

- Palliation (See Chapter 12 for further discussion.)

Radiation Therapy for Primary Breast Cancer

- Increased percentage of early-stage disease with smaller primary tumors
- More breast-preserving options for women with early stage I and II breast cancers; however, fewer than 50% of women with stage I and II breast cancer in the United States are treated with XRT.
- Improved radiation equipment, techniques, and procedures
- Wider availability of XRT facilities
- Benefits of XRT

  Improved cosmetic outcome

  Consideration of psychological and sexual concerns

  Equivalent to mastectomy for local control of disease
- Contraindications to XRT (Morrow & Harris, 2004)

  Patients who are in first or second trimester of pregnancy

  Two or more primary tumors in separate quadrants of the breast

  Diffuse microcalcifications within the breast

  Previous XRT to the same breast

  Persistent positive-tissue margins after surgery
- Relative contraindications

  History of collagen vascular disease (e.g., scleroderma, active lupus erythematosus)

  Multiple gross tumors in same breast quadrant

> *Presence of a large tumor in a small breast will limit the cosmetic outcome*
>
> *Large breast size*

- Goals of BCS and XRT

  1. Achieve survival equivalent to that of a mastectomy

  2. Maintain local control and low rate of recurrence in the breast

  3. Preserve cosmetic outcome for the patient

- Patient selection for XRT must take into account:

  History and physical examination

  Mammographic evaluation

  Histologic assessment

  Patient needs and expectations

- Procedure

  BCS to excise gross tumor (e.g., excisional biopsy or lumpectomy) with clear margin of surrounding normal tissue

  Technical aspects related to lumpectomy include:

  1. Surgical incision directly over area of tumor

  2. Curvilinear or transverse incision when tumors are located in upper part of breast

  3. Preservation of subcutaneous fat and avoidance of skin flaps

  Re-excision is indicated in the presence of positive tumor margins and unknown histologic margins of resection at initial surgery.

XRT to entire breast to eradicate microscopic residual disease

- Risk factors for recurrence after BCS and XRT (Morrow & Harris, 2004)

  Young age is associated with increased risk of local recurrence and worse outcome after mastectomy.

  Extensive intraductal component when margins of resection are not evaluated.

  Extent of resection using incisional biopsy is higher than with excisional biopsy.

  Use of adjuvant systemic therapy decreases the rate of local recurrence.

Postmastectomy Radiation Therapy

- Postmastectomy XRT is the use of radiation to the chest and draining lymph nodes as adjuvant treatment after mastectomy.
- Indications for use of postoperative radiation

  1. Reduces rate of local-regional tumor recurrence (in chest wall, axilla, internal mammary, or supraclavicular lymph nodes).

  2. Improves survival by eradicating residual local disease that is the only site of persistent cancer after mastectomy and a potential source of distant metastasis or "seeding."

- Patients with four or more positive nodes or an advanced primary tumor benefit from postmastectomy radiation XRT (Wong & Harris, 2004).

• XRT should not be given concurrently with anthracycline-containing chemotherapy.

Steps in the Radiation Treatment Process

• Prior to starting radiation treatment, several steps must be completed.

1. Pretreatment consultation

   Ideally, consultation occurs after diagnosis and before any local or systemic therapy is initiated.

   It includes discussion of the specific role of XRT in the overall breast cancer treatment plan.

   During consultation, a physical examination is conducted, diagnostic studies are performed, and the radiation oncologist reviews the pathology.

2. Treatment planning

   Once a decision is made to include XRT, the treatment planning session is initiated.

   Treatment planning is also called a "simulation" procedure.

   Goals of treatment planning are to maximize the radiation dose to the specific treatment area and minimize the dose to other normal tissues, such as the lung and heart.

• Treatment-planning procedure

   Takes approximately 1 hour

   Radiation therapists and radiation oncologists measure the breast and axilla.

A series of X-rays are done on the simulation-planning machine to delineate the breast and draining lymph node areas.

Skin surface markings are made to serve as landmarks for treatment.

Immobilization devices made of Styrofoam casts are made to help ensure consistent patient positioning for daily radiation treatments.

- Patient teaching before treatment planning

The experience may be uncomfortable.

Convey to the patient that the focus is on careful and detailed measurement.

Questions or concerns can be addressed before or after treatment planning.

After treatment planning is complete, the patient will receive an appointment to start daily XRT.

Daily Radiation Therapy Treatment

- XRT consists of two components:
  1. External beam radiation to the primary tumor
  2. Electron treatment or radiation implant to boost the site of the original tumor

- External beam radiation

High-energy photons are emitted from a linear accelerator.

Radiation fields cover the entire breast, the underlying chest wall, and the lower axilla, using opposing tangential fields to minimize lung and heart exposure.

A third anterior field may be added if the upper axillary and supraclavicular areas are included.

Whole-breast XRT dose ranges from 46 to 50 Gy.

The typical daily dose is 180 to 200 cGy delivered 5 days a week over a 4.5- to 5-week period.

- Radiation boost to excision site

The goal is to increase the local control to the primary tumor site without decreasing cosmetic outcome.

Procedure

1. Outpatient treatment after completion of XRT to whole breast.

2. Electron beam penetrates tissue to a specific depth, allowing treatment of the tumor bed and sparing underlying lungs and ribs from radiation.

3. Treatment takes an additional five to eight daily fractions of 200 cGy.

4. Boosts total dose to the primary tumor site to 60 cGy or higher.

- Radiation implant

Interstitial implantation of radioactive Iridium-192

Used as an alternative when boost treatment cannot be accomplished using electrons

1. Less frequently used method for radiation boost today

2. Invasive procedure requiring a 2- to 3-day hospital stay

- Nursing care during radiation implant

  Manage mild discomfort associated with the procedure

  Reinforce necessity of radiation safety precautions for patient with nursing staff, family members, and visitors

  Provide emotional support to the patient during the isolation period

Patient and Family Education During the Radiation Therapy (Perun, 2004)

- Goals
  1. Prepare the patient for the course of XRT.
  2. Teach the patient about potential side effects.
  3. Help coordinate patient care activities during the radiation treatment experience.

- Prepare for a radiation treatment.

  Describe the radiation treatment course. "Walk" the patient through a treatment.

  Explain the rationale for the total number of treatments needed and what patients can expect to hear and see in the treatment room.

  Reassure the patient that she will not feel discomfort during the actual treatment.

  Reassure the patient that radiation therapists will work closely with her during her therapy.

  Time spent in radiation treatment room (15 minutes) is used to set up accurate positioning.

  Actual treatment time is approximately 3 minutes.

Side Effects of Radiation Therapy for Primary Breast Cancer

- Table 8-1 lists the side effects of radiation therapy to the breast or chest wall.

- Acute and late effects

  Acute side effects occur during treatment and up to 6 months post-XRT.

  Late effects occur after 6 months (reader is referred to Chapter 14 for a discussion of late effects of XRT).

- Common acute side effects

  Skin reactions

  Arm and breast edema

  Intermittent aches and pains in the treated breast, chest wall, or axilla

  Fatigue

- Teaching points about side effects:

  1. Emphasize local versus systemic effects of XRT.

  2. Reassure patients that they will not become radioactive.

  3. Teach patients that they will not experience severe skin "burns."

  4. Clarify information, dispel misconceptions, and identify fears about radiation as a treatment modality.

TABLE 8-1
Potential Acute Side Effects of Radiation Therapy to Breast/Chest Wall

Side Effect	Average Onset	Usual Duration	Appearance/ Presentation	Intervention
Skin erythema	Approximately 2 weeks after start of treatment.	Resolution usually within 10 to 14 days after end of treatment.	Variable. Mild redness to brisk or bright redness. Mild to moderate discomfort.	Unscented hydrophilic creams such as Aquaphor, Eucerin, Lubriderm. Unscented, 99–100% pure aloe vera gel (no added perfumes, colors). Avoid tight bras, underwire bras.
Hyperpigmentation	Approximately 2 weeks after start of treatment. May be more pronounced in darker pigmented women.	Resolves slowly after end of treatment. Mild hyper-pigmentation may last for months.	Presents as mild to deep tanning of the skin. May be associated with mild discomfort.	As above.

| Itching/folliculitis (Irritation of hair follicles) | Approximately 10 to 14 days after start of treatment. | Variable—may start to resolve at end of treatment course to entire breast (before start of boost treatment); usually much improved by end of treatment course. | Itchy skin appears slightly red and dry. Folliculitis appears as small red dots often in sternal, infraclavicular, and supraclavicular area. Occasionally found on back below clavicle 20 exit dose. May cause mild discomfort and itching. | Oatmeal colloidal-based soaps (such as Aveeno). Make paste and apply to affected area, let dry for 3–5 minutes and rinse off with cool water. Oatmeal colloidal-based bath products may be added to bath. 99–100% pure aloe vera gel (no added dyes or perfumes). Unscented hydrophilic creams such as those listed for erythema. Diphenhydramine—25 mg may be taken at night for severe itching. |

(*continues*)

TABLE 8-1 (*continued*)
Potential Acute Side Effects of Radiation Therapy to Breast/Chest Wall

Side Effect	Average Onset	Usual Duration	Appearance/ Presentation	Intervention
Fatigue	Highly variable approximately 2–3 weeks after start of treatment. May be an increased effect with previous or concurrent chemotherapy.	May last up to 2–3 weeks after end of radiation treatments. Average is 10 to 14 days. May be prolonged if receiving chemotherapy.	Increased tiredness late afternoon or early evening. Most women are able to continue their usual routines.	Earlier bedtime; late afternoon or early evening rest period. Good nutrition—avoid dieting during course of treatment. Conserve energy by having family and friends help as needed. Moderate exercise such as walking has been found to help energy levels.

Dry desquamation (dry peeling)	Approximately 3 weeks after starting radiation.	Usually resolves within 2 weeks of finishing radiation treatments.	Dry flaking or peeling of skin frequently associated with erythema or hyperpigmentation of skin.	Use of highly moisturizing hydrophilic creams such as Aquaphor and Eucerin.
Moist desquamation (moist peeling)	4–5 weeks after start of radiation therapy.	Usually completely healed within 2–3 weeks after end of radiation treatments.	Moist peeling of the skin with associated erythema. Area may ooze or weep. May be associated with mild to moderate discomfort depending on severity of reaction. Increased reaction is possible if patient receiving concurrent chemotherapy. Often occurs in	Gentle rinsing with drying antibacterial solutions such as Hibiclens/chlorhexidine gluconate or 1/4-1/2 strength H_2O_2. Pat dry with soft clean towel 2–3 times a day. This can be followed by application of unscented hydrophilic cream such as Aquaphor, followed by nonadherent dressing such as

(continues)

TABLE 8-1 (*continued*)
Potential Acute Side Effects of Radiation Therapy to Breast/Chest Wall

Side Effect	Average Onset	Usual Duration	Appearance/ Presentation	Intervention
			areas with increased shearing friction such as inframammary fold and axilla.	Aquaphor gauze, covered with a soft ABD pad and held in place by a bra or large size body netting. Moist soaks can be used such as aluminum acetate solutions: Bluboro and Domeboro for 20 minutes 3 times a day. Moisture vapor permeable dressing may be used such as Opsite, although they can be difficult to adhere in skin folds.

Intermittent aches and pains in breast	May occur approximately 1 week after start of radiation.	Can persist for months after radiation finishes although usually with decreased frequency.	Patients often describe pain as intermittent sharp twinge in the breast.	Avoid use of tape on irritated skin. Can use gentle luke-warm shower spray to help debride skin. Allow area to be open to air whenever possible. If pain is moderate or severe, use of NSAID or mild narcotic may be indicated. Reassure that this is a normal occurrence and may be alleviated with use of NSAID.
Breast edema	As above.	Can persist for months after radiation.	Slight to moderate swelling of treated breast. Breast may feel full or heavy.	As above. Wearing a supportive bra may improve comfort.

(continues)

TABLE 8-1 *(continued)*
Potential Acute Side Effects of Radiation Therapy to Breast/Chest Wall

Side Effect	Average Onset	Usual Duration	Appearance/ Presentation	Intervention
Hair loss in treatment portal (fine hair of breast, nipple, and possibly small amount of axillary hair)	Usually starts 3–4 weeks at doses of 30–35 Gy.	Variable. May take 1–6 months for hair to grow back.	Typically not very noticeable or bothersome to patients except when associated with folliculitis or itching.	Follow interventions for itching/ folliculitis.

Source: Perun, J., 2004. Reprinted with permission.

Skin Reactions (Porock, et al., 1998; Sitton, 1992a)

- Erythema or redness

  May occur immediately after first radiation treatment

  Generally dose dependent and increases throughout the course of XRT

  Higher risk for fair-skinned individuals

  Increase in redness also heightened along a bony prominence, such as the clavicle

- Increased pigmentation

  Skin reaction is dose dependent and most often occurs in darker pigmented individuals.

  Pigmentation appears as series of dark dots in the treatment field.

- Folliculitis with pruritus

  Skin reaction is dose dependent.

  Mild emollient or lotion will help decrease itchiness.

  Oatmeal-based soap applied to the skin may help relieve itchiness.

  Areas of higher risk include the skin folds and general breast area.

- Hair loss in the treated area (reaction is temporary)

- Dry desquamation (dry peeling)

  Most commonly seen in areas of bony prominence, such as the clavicle.

  Mild emollient placed on the skin after treatment will help soothe the irritated area.

- Moist desquamation (moist peeling)

  Skin reaction is dose dependent and most often occurs with concurrent chemotherapy.

  Rarely occurs without concurrent chemotherapy.

  Several skin-care guidelines are available to manage moist reactions.

  May require a radiation treatment break if the moist reaction is severe.

- Factors influencing skin reactions

  Skin folds (i.e., inframammary and axilla) included in the radiation treatment field

  Older age

  Concurrent use of topical steroids near the XRT field

  Higher radiation dose fraction and higher total radiation dose

  Enhanced skin effects in electron beam boost

  Enhanced skin reactions, with chest wall radiation occurring at the XRT beam exit site in the upper back

- Management of skin reactions (Sitton, 1992b)

  Majority of skin-care regimens for patients receiving breast irradiation are nonresearch based.

  Recommendations depend on what has worked most effectively in clinical practice and on institutional policies (see Table 8-2).

TABLE 8-2

General Skin-Care Guidelines for Radiation Treatment to the Breast and Chest Wall

General precare guidelines are as follows:
1. Keep breast or chest wall clean and dry.
2. Cleanse the treated area with gentle soap (e.g., Ivory, Basis, Pears, Neutrogena, or unscented Dove).
3. Avoid the use of creams, lotions, perfumes, or deodorant in the treatment area unless directed by a radiation oncologist, nurse, or radiation therapist.
4. Avoid extremes of temperature, such as heating pads, hot-water bottles, and ice packs in the treatment area. Avoid hot tubs and saunas.
5. Avoid excess friction or rubbing.
6. Do not wear tight clothing or an underwire bra; use a sports bra during XRT.
7. Use an electric razor to shave under the treated arm.
8. Protect the skin in the treatment field from exposure to direct sunlight by either covering the skin or using a sunblock with SPF of 15 or higher.

General aftercare instructions include the following:
1. Occasional aches and pains in the treated breast and chest wall may continue for weeks or months after finishing XRT. Use an NSAID such as ibuprofen.
2. Skin changes will gradually improve over the 1 to 2 weeks following completion of treatment. The treated skin may look tanned.
3. The breast tissue may feel thicker and firmer after XRT. Continue self-breast examinations monthly in order to remain familiar with the feel of the breast tissue.
4. Call the oncology team with any concerns or questions.
5. The skin may feel dry after radiation therapy. Use a skin moisturizer for at least 2 weeks after the end of radiation treatment.

(continues)

TABLE 8-2 (*continued*)
General Skin-Care Guidelines for Radiation Treatment to the Breast and Chest Wall

6. If previously irradiated skin is exposed to direct sunlight, cover or protect with SPF 15 or higher.
7. If any areas of redness, heat, or swelling develop in the treated breast, hand, or arm, call the health care provider.

The following information should be included if patients have had an axillary dissection and/or XRT to the axilla:

8. Wear gloves when gardening or using harsh chemicals such as bleach.
9. For an extended period of time, avoid using the affected arm or hand to carry heavy packages.
10. If you get a cut or burn on the affected arm or hand, gently cleanse the area and apply antibacterial cream.
11. Use the untreated arm for blood drawing, blood pressures, and vaccinations and/or injections.

Arm and Breast Edema

- Arm edema or lymphedema occurs most often in patients receiving XRT to the axilla after axillary dissection.

- Etiology is not well understood but is related to obliteration of lymphatics in the axilla by surgery and XRT.

- The reader is referred to Chapter 16 for a more detailed discussion about lymphedema.

- Breast edema occurs as mild breast discomfort and feelings of fullness in the treated breast.

- Arm and breast edema may occur shortly after radiation is complete or within the first year after XRT.
- Breast edema may take up to several months to resolve.

  Breast edema may be treated with nonsteroidal anti-inflammatory drugs.

  Symptomatic relief using cotton sport bras helps alleviate heaviness and discomfort.

Intermittent Twinges and Shooting Pains

- These may occur in the treated breast, chest wall, or axilla.
- These are common and normal after surgery and radiation therapy.
- Treat them with mild analgesics.
- Twinges may last for several months to years after treatment ends.

Fatigue

- This is a very common reaction experienced by patients receiving XRT.
- Mechanisms of radiation-related fatigue are not well understood.
- Most likely a multifactorial etiology:

  Recovery from recent surgery

  Previous or concurrent chemotherapy

  Increased tumor burden

Concurrent medications, such as antiemetics or analgesics

Nutritional deficit

Demands of daily treatment in the radiation oncology department for a period of 5 to 6 weeks

No corresponding decrease in family and work responsibilities during XRT

Presence of other symptom clusters, such as sleeplessness and restlessness and anxiety over disease and treatment

Interventions for fatigue (See Chapter 15 for further discussion of cancer-related fatigue.)

Emotional Response During Radiation Therapy

- Patients may experience many emotional reactions during the course of XRT. Emotional reactions may not necessarily be related directly to radiation but to the experience of having breast cancer. In addition, there may be an age-related emotional response to treatment (Dow & Lafferty, 2000). Thus, it is important for the radiation oncology nurse to

  1. Assess the patient's psychosocial status before treatment and regularly during XRT.

  2. Suggest the availability of support groups, discussion groups, and community resources, and refer as needed.

  3. Discuss other psychosocial interventions available (Kolcaba & Fox, 1999).

  4. Provide a number for patients to call and speak directly to a nurse for questions or concerns.

REFERENCES

Dow, K. H., & Lafferty, P. (2000). Quality of life, survivorship, and psychosocial adjustment of young women with breast cancer after breast-conserving surgery and radiation therapy. *Oncology Nursing Forum, 27*, 1555–1564.

Kolcaba, K., & Fox, C. (1999). The effects of guided imagery on comfort of women with early stage breast cancer undergoing radiation therapy. *Oncology Nursing Forum, 26*, 67–72.

Morrow, M., & Harris, J. R. (2004). Local management of invasive breast cancer. In J. R. Harris, M. Lippman, M. Morrow, & C. K. Osborne (Eds.), *Diseases of the breast* (3rd ed., pp. 720–744). Philadelphia: Lippincott Williams & Wilkins.

Perun, J. (2004). Radiation therapy. In K. H. Dow (Ed.), *Contemporary issues in breast cancer* (2nd ed., pp. 110–133). Sudbury, MA: Jones and Bartlett.

Porock, D., Kristjanson, L., Nikoletti, S., Cameron, F., & Pedler, P. (1998). Predicting the severity of radiation skin reactions in women with breast cancer. *Oncology Nursing Forum, 25*, 1019–1029.

Sitton, E. (1992a). Early and late radiation-induced skin alterations Part I: Mechanisms of skin changes. *Oncology Nursing Forum, 19*, 801–807.

Sitton, E. (1992b). Early and late radiation-induced skin alterations Part II: Nursing care of irradiated skin. *Oncology Nursing Forum, 25*, 907–912.

Wong, J., & Harris, J. R. (2004). Postmastectomy radiation therapy. In J. R. Harris (Ed.), *Diseases of the breast* (3rd ed., pp. 785–799). Philadelphia: Lippincott Williams & Wilkins.

CHAPTER NINE

Adjuvant Chemotherapy

Introduction

- Adjuvant systemic therapy is recommended for women with invasive disease.

- Adjuvant systemic therapy is the administration of chemotherapy or endocrine therapy after primary treatment to reduce the risk of recurrence. The focus of this chapter is the use of adjuvant chemotherapy (Stearns & Davidson, 2004).

- Chemotherapy and dosing strategies are constantly changing. A brief history of the role of adjuvant chemotherapy is outlined in Table 9-1.

Adjuvant Chemotherapy Principles

- National Comprehensive Cancer Network (NCCN) guidelines for the adjuvant treatment of breast cancer with chemotherapy can be accessed online at www.nccn.org/professionals/physician_gls/PDF/breast.pdf.

TABLE 9-1

Historical Perspective in the Use of Adjuvant Chemotherapy

1960–1970s	Postoperative adjuvant chemotherapy used in patients with involved lymph nodes
1980s	Doxorubicin-based chemotherapy trials
	Clinical trials chemotherapy in patients without axillary nodal involvement
	Combined chemoendocrine therapy
1990s	High-dose chemotherapy with autologous bone marrow transplantation declined
	Neoadjuvant chemotherapy
	Taxanes in adjuvant setting
2000s	Dose-dense chemotherapy
	Targeted therapy

- In general, adjuvant chemotherapy may be indicated for women with lymph node–positive disease or in women with high-risk, lymph node–negative breast cancer (Davidson & Osborne, 2004).

- Chemotherapy is given with more than one chemotherapeutic agent over a 3- to 6-month period of time.

- Anthracycline-containing regimens are more effective than regimens that do not contain anthracycline (e.g., CMF), but there is greater toxicity with anthracyclines.

- Women with node-positive disease may also benefit from the addition of a taxane to the chemotherapy regimen.

- Several randomized clinical trials have not shown benefit with the use of increased dose intensity with colony-stimulating factor.

- Dose-dense chemotherapy is the administration of chemotherapy within the shortest period of time between cycles to allow for the maximal drug effect on tumor growth suggest benefit.

- Women with receptor-positive disease may benefit from endocrine therapy after chemotherapy. The reader is referred to Chapter 11 for a more thorough discussion of hormonal/endocrine therapy.

- Preoperative or neoadjuvant chemotherapy is the use of systemic therapy before surgery. It is generally used for women with larger T3 or T4 lesions with the goal of reducing the tumor size to increase the likelihood of women receiving breast conserving surgery.

- Randomized clinical trials are evaluating the effectiveness of trastuzumab in combination with chemotherapy for women with high-risk, early stage HER-2 overexpressing breast cancer. Currently, trastuzumab is not part of standard treatment in the adjuvant setting.

Adjuvant Chemotherapy Regimens

- Table 9-2 outlines chemotherapy commonly used for breast cancer and includes: cyclophosphamide, doxorubicin, epirubicin, paclitaxel, docetaxel, 5-fluorouracil, and methotrexate.

TABLE 9-2
Adjuvant Chemotherapy

Cyclophosphamide (Cytoxan)

Mechanism of action	Alkylating agent that causes cross-linking of DNA strands that prevent DNA synthesis and cell division
Indications/Use	Adjuvant therapy
Toxicity	Nausea and vomiting
	Alopecia
	Urotoxicity, hemorrhagic cystitis
	Myelosuppression

Doxorubicin

Mechanism of action	Antitumor antibiotic that binds directly to DNA base pairs and inhibits DNA and RNA synthesis
Indications/Use	Adjuvant therapy
	Advanced disease
Special precautions	Maximum cumulative lifetime dose is 450–550 mg/m2
	<400 mg/m2 cumulative lifetime dose recommended in patients who have had prior cardiotoxic regimens or chest radiation
	Vesicant

Toxicity	Cardiotoxicity
	Nausea and vomiting
	Myelosuppression
	Alopecia
	Stomatitis

Epirubicin (EPI)

Mechanism of action	DNA-strand breakage mediated by anthracycline effects on topoisomerase II
Indications/Use	Adjuvant therapy
	Advanced disease
Special precautions	Vesicant
	Administer through sidearm of freely flowing IV infusion
	Lifetime cumulative dose of 900–1000 mg/m2
	Reduce dose in patients with prior chest radiation or anthracycline
Toxicity	Myelosuppression: dose-limiting leukopenia
	Nausea and vomiting: common
	Stomatitis: dose dependent
	Alopecia

(continues)

TABLE 9-2 (*continued*)
Adjuvant Chemotherapy

	Cardiac effects: potentially irreversible congestive heart failure
	Red-orange discoloration of urine
	Diarrhea: occasional
Paclitaxel	
Mechanism of action	Enhanced formation and stabilization of microtubules
Indications/Use	Adjuvant therapy
	Advanced disease
Special precautions	Hypersensitivity reaction minimized with pretreatment of: dexamethasone 20 mg orally or intravenously 12 hours and 6 hours prior to infusion, diphenhydramine 50 mg IV and cimetidine 300 mg IV 30 minutes prior to infusion
	Mixed in containers that do NOT contain polyvinylchloride or diethylhexlphtalate (DEHP) plastics
	Use an in-line filter
	Do not administer if patient has known sensitivity to Cremophor EL
	ANC should be >1500 prior to initial or subsequent doses of paclitaxel
	Avoid concomitant use of ketoconazole
	Cardiac monitoring if history of conduction abnormalities

Toxicity	First hour of infusion, take vital signs every 15 minutes; second hour of infusion, take vital signs every 30 minutes; or per hospital policy
	Dose limiting: neutropenia, mucositis (with longer infusion), neurotoxicity
	Frequent: myalgias, arthralgias, alopecia
	Rare: thrombocytopenia, anemia, nausea and vomiting, diarrhea
	Hypersensitivity reaction (dyspnea, hypotension, bronchospasm, urticaria may result from Cremophor)

5-fluorouracil

Mechanism of action	Pyrimidine antimetabolite; inhibit the formation of thymidine synthetase needed for DNA synthesis
Indications/Use	Adjuvant therapy
Toxicity	Neutropenia and thrombocytopenia
	Cutaneous effects in nails, skin, and hair loss
	Nausea and vomiting

Methotrexate

Mechanism of action	Antimetabolite, folic acid antagonist; blocks the enzyme dihyrofolate reductase that inhibits conversion of folic acid to tetrahydrofolic acid. Inhibits precursors of DNA, RNA, and cellular proteins
Indications/Use	Adjuvant therapy

(continues)

TABLE 9-2 (*continued*)
Adjuvant Chemotherapy

Toxicity	Stomatitis
	Diarrhea
	Nausea and vomiting
Docetaxel (Taxotere)	
Mechanism of action	Inhibits mitotic spindle apparatus by enhanced formation and stabilization of microtubules
Special precautions	Severe hypersensitivity reactions (flushing, hypotension, dyspnea) can be minimized with premedication of dexamethasone 8 mg PO BID for 5 days starting 1 day before docetaxel
	Should not infuse through polyvinyl chloride (PVC) tubing
Toxicity	Myelosuppression common and dose limiting
	Hypersensitivity reaction uncommon
	Alopecia, skin, and nail changes
	Nausea and vomiting: common and brief
	Mild mucositis
	Fluid retention common
	Fatigue, myalgias common
	Mild sensorimotor neuropathy

- Standard adjuvant chemotherapy regimens include:

    CMF (cyclophosphamide/methotrexate, fluorouracil)

    FAC (fluorouracil/doxorubicin/cyclophosphamide)

    AC (doxorubicin/cyclophosphamide)

    *AC (doxorubicin/cyclophosphamide) + sequential pacli-
    taxel*

    CEF (cyclophosphamide/epirubicin/fluorouracil)

- Side effect management of chemotherapy is contained in Chapter 10.

Support for Decision Making in Adjuvant Chemotherapy (National Institutes of Health, 2000)

- Patients need time to discuss and share their concerns in making decisions about chemotherapy.
  Effective communication between the oncology team
  and the patient is critical. The following are points to
  consider in helping to support patients in their decision making:

    *Clarify their concerns and help evaluate the risks and ben-
    efits with treatment.*

    *Discuss how their treatment may alter their lifestyle and
    daily routines.*

    Explain the range of treatment side effects and management.

    *Explore the impact of the treatment on their personal
    quality of life.*

    Discuss their concerns about clinical trials.

REFERENCES

Davidson, N., & Osborne, C. (2004). Adjuvant systemic therapy treatment guidelines. In J. R. Harris, M. E. Lippman, M. Morrow, & C. K. Osborne (Eds.), *Diseases of the breast* (3rd ed., pp. 945–947). Philadelphia: Lippincott Williams & Wilkins.

National Institutes of Health. (2000). *NIH consensus development conference statement on adjuvant therapy for breast cancer.* Retrieved October 22, 2004, from http://consensus.nih.gov.

Stearns, V., & Davidson, N. E. (2004). Adjuvant chemotherapy and chemoendocrine therapy. In J. R. Harris, M. E. Lippman, M. Morrow, & C. K. Osborne (Eds.), *Diseases of the breast* (3rd ed., pp. 893–919). Philadelphia: Lippincott Williams & Wilkins.

CHAPTER TEN

Symptom Management of Acute Side Effects of Adjuvant Chemotherapy

Adjuvant Chemotherapy: Acute Side Effects
(Geddie, 2004)

- Acute side effects of adjuvant chemotherapy are well known, expected, and can be managed through a coordinated patient-centered team approach.

- The severity of side effects varies among individuals and is related to several factors such as type of adjuvant regimen and degree of supportive care.

- Modifications in normal lifestyle and routine may be needed during chemotherapy.

Nursing Roles in Side Effect Management

- Educate the patient and family.

- Provide emotional support for the patient and family.
- Coordinate patient care.
- Facilitate support groups.
- Manage the side effects of treatment.

Common Toxicity Related to Treatment

- Neutropenia
- Alopecia or hair loss
- Nausea and vomiting
- Thromboembolic events
- Weight gain
- Mucositis
- Fatigue
- Arthralgia/myalgia
- Toxicity is graded on a scale from 0 to 4 based on criteria of the National Cancer Institute

Neutropenia (Wujcik, 2004)

- Definition: Reduction in the number of circulating neutrophils to less than $1,000/\mu L$.
- Grade 3 and 4 neutropenia increases risk of life-threatening infection.
- Neutropenia is the largest predictor of infection in patients with cancer.

- Absolute neutrophil count (ANC) is calculated by the following formula:

  segmented neutrophils (%) + bands (%) × white blood cell count = ANC

- Severity

  ANC >1,500/μL = Grade 1 (slight)

  ANC 1000–1490/μL = Grade 2 (mild)

  ANC 999–500/μL = Grade 3 (moderate)

  ANC <500/μL = Grade 4 (severe)

- Common Toxicity Criteria of the National Cancer Institute provide a set of measures of commonly experienced side effects of clinical trials to help decrease the subjectivity of measurement (Table 10-1).

TABLE 10-1
Common Toxicity Criteria of the National Cancer Institute

Grade 0	Grade 1	Grade 2	Grade 3	Grade 4
Normal	ANC >1.5	ANC <1.0	ANC <0.5	ANC <0.1

- Short-term neutropenia lasts less than a week.
- Long-term neutropenia exceeds 1 to 2 weeks.
- Risk factors include advancing age, concurrent or prior radiation therapy, history of febrile neutropenia, and poor nutritional status.
- Chemotherapy agents, when used in combination for breast cancer will increase risk of neutropenia.

These agents include doxorubicin, cyclophos-phamide, paclitaxel, and methotrexate.

- Neutropenic episodes during chemotherapy are pre-dictable, with the nadir (or lowest) white blood count occurring 10 to 14 days after treatment, with full recovery 3 to 4 weeks after treatment.

- Signs and symptoms

  Fever with temperature higher than 38ºC or 100.4ºF in a 24-hour period or temperature spike of 38.5ºC or 101.3ºF

  Pain and tenderness

  Change in character or color of urine, sputum, or stool

  Breaks in skin integrity

  Dysuria or frequency of urination

  Malaise, lethargy, myalgia

  In moderate to severe neutropenia, objective signs of infec-tion are generally absent due to lack of circulating neutrophils.

- Management of neutropenia

  Prompt recognition and work-up for suspected area of infection.

  Physical assessment, blood cultures, chest radiograph (CXR), and other studies as needed.

  Hematopoietic growth factors decrease the severity of neutropenia.

  Granulocyte colony-stimulating factor (G-CSF) is FDA agent approved for chemotherapy-induced neutropenia (CIN). Agents include filgrastim and pegfilgrastim.

Randomized clinical trials demonstrate comparable safety and efficacy between daily injection of filgrastim and fixed doses of pegfilgrastim.

High-risk patients may receive prophylactic G-CSF therapy.

Antibiotic, antiviral, and/or antifungal therapy may be indicated.

- Patient self-care management

  Monitor temperature at least twice daily.

  Use steps to decrease colonization, such as dietary changes and avoidance of individuals with known or suspected infections.

  Practice good skin and self-care hygiene.

  Implement precautions to reduce risk of upper respiratory infection.

- Management guidelines for fever and neutropenia developed by the NCCN can be accessed online at www.nccn.org/professionals/physician_gls/PDF/fever.pdf.

Hair Loss (Reeves, 2004)

- Although most discussions of hair loss focus on scalp hair, there is also loss of hair in the axilla, pubis, eyebrows, and eyelashes.

- Degrees of hair loss

  Total hair loss occurs with doxorubicin.

  High potential for hair loss or alopecia occurs with cyclophosphamide and paclitaxel.

Moderate potential for hair loss occurs with methotrexate and 5-fluorouracil (5-FU).

Hair thinning and moderate hair loss occur with cyclophosphamide, methotrexate, and 5-fluorouracil (CMF).

- Hair loss typically begins around 2 to 3 weeks after first exposure to chemotherapy, with continued loss over 3 to 4 weeks.

- Differences in the rate of hair loss can occur.

  Hair loss with paclitaxel occurs around 2 to 3 weeks and may be sudden and cumulative.

- Common toxicity criteria of the NCI for hair loss is listed on Table 10-2.

TABLE 10-2
Common Toxicity Criteria of the National Cancer Institute

Grade 0	Grade 1	Grade 2	Grade 3	Grade 4
Normal	Mild hair loss	Pronounced hair loss	—	—

- Hair loss management focuses on preparatory information.

  Help the patient anticipate hair loss and prepare for it.

  Obtain a wig to fit normal hair color and style prior to the beginning of chemotherapy.

  Suggest turbans and hats to protect the scalp during chemotherapy.

Access the services of the ACS "Look Good . . . Feel Better" Program for community information and support.

Suggest cutting the hair to a manageable style before chemotherapy begins.

Use a mild shampoo and conditioner.

Avoid electric curlers and curling irons.

Avoid excessive hair brushing.

When hair loss begins, it may occur in a rapid manner, or the hair may thin over time.

The scalp and skin around the ears may become itchy and dry, requiring mild soap and soothing emollients or lotions.

- Hair loss is temporary, and regrowth may be seen 3 months after completion of chemotherapy.

  The new hair color may differ from the original color.

  Hair texture also may differ from that of the original hair (may be softer and finer).

- Reeves (2004) provides an excellent assessment and management algorithm for alopecia.

Nausea and Vomiting (Wickham, 2004)

- The major goal is prevention of nausea and vomiting.
- Chemotherapy agents are categorized in order from high to minimal emetogenicity.
  1. Level 5—High
  2. Level 3–4—Moderate

    3.   Level 2—Low

    4.   Level 1—Minimal

- Doxorubicin, epirubicin, cyclophosphamide (oral and intravenous), fluorouracil, and paclitaxel doses used in breast cancer treatment are considered moderate to moderately high emetogenic agents.

- Patient characteristics that place them at risk for nausea and vomiting include female gender, younger age, and a history of motion sickness or hyperemesis in pregnancy.

- Patients at lower risk for nausea and vomiting are those with a history of chronic, daily, high alcohol intake.

- Incidence and severity of nausea and vomiting are influenced by many factors including specific chemotherapeutic agent, dose, schedule and route of administration, and patient characteristics.

- The NCI grading criteria for nausea and vomiting is listed in Table 10-3.

- Pathophysiology of nausea and vomiting

  Vomiting results from the central stimulation of the brain's vomiting center and chemoreceptor trigger zone (CTZ).

  Peripheral stimulation of enterochromaffin cells in the gastrointestinal (GI) tract.

- Classification of nausea and vomiting are in Table 10-4.

TABLE 10-3
Common Toxicity Criteria for Nausea and Vomiting

	Grade 0	Grade 1	Grade 2	Grade 3	Grade 4
Nausea	None	Able to eat reasonable intake	Intake significantly decreased but can eat	No significant intake	>10 episodes in 24 hours
Vomiting	None	One episode in 24 hours	2–5 episodes in 24 hours	6–10 episodes in 24 hours	Requiring parenteral support

TABLE 10-4
Classification of Nausea and Vomiting

Acute	Delayed	Anticipatory	Refractory
Occurs within 24 hours of chemotherapy	Occurs after 24 hours after chemotherapy and lasts up to 5 days	Occurs before chemotherapy and is related to poor nausea and vomiting control during prior treatment	Unresponsive to antiemetic therapy

- Principles for the management of emetogenic chemotherapy regimens developed by the NCCN can be accessed online at www.nccn.org/professionals/physician_gls/PDF/antiemesis.pdf.

Types of Antiemetics
- $5-HT_3$ receptor antagonists
- Dopamine receptor antagonists
- Corticosteroids
- Benzodiazepines
  Used for anticipatory nausea and vomiting and anxiety

Serotonin Antagonists
- Wide use of $5-HT_3$ receptor serotonin antagonists (e.g., ondansetron, granisetron, dolasetron, and palonosetron) have reduced experience of acute nausea and vomiting.
- Granisetron, ondansetron, dolasetron, and palonosetron provide equivalent protection for moderately to highly emetogenic drugs.
- $5-HT_3$ receptor antagonists bind to serotonin receptors on the afferent vagus and splanchnic nerves in the GI tract and CTZ for about 24 hours.
- These agents work within the vomiting center of the brain and on the enterochromaffin cells in the gut.
- These agents are first-line therapy for moderately to highly emetogenic chemotherapy.

- Palonosetron became available in November 2003. It is a pharmacologically distinct 5-HT$_3$ antagonists having about 100-fold higher binding affinity for the 5-HT$_3$ receptor compared to the other serotonin antagonists.

- Other than palonosetron, 5-HT$_3$ agents are not as effective for control of delayed nausea and vomiting.

  Side effects include headache, constipation, lightheadedness, and sedation.

Dopamine Receptor Antagonists

- Metoclopramide, phenothiazines, and butyrophenones bind to dopamine receptors and block impulses from the vomiting center.

- These agents are used to treat nausea and vomiting from low to moderate emetogenic chemotherapy and delayed nausea and vomiting.

- Major disadvantage is that these agents cause extrapyramidal reactions, with the most common symptom called *akathisia* or dancing leg syndrome.

Corticosteroids

- Mechanism of action as an antiemetic is unknown, but corticosteroids have both central and peripheral effects. They also may decrease the capillary permeability of CNS.

- Increases anti-emetic effect of 5-HT$_3$ by 20%.

- Useful for delayed nausea and vomiting.

- Insomnia is a bothersome side effect.

Benzodiazepines

- These have a modest antiemetic effect and are thus combined with other antiemetics.
- The mechanism of antiemetic action is unknown.
- Lorazepam decreases anxiety and agitation and may alter the perception of nausea and vomiting.
- Lorazepam may be used to minimize anticipatory nausea and vomiting.

Complementary Interventions

- Behavioral interventions:

  Guided imagery, hypnosis, relaxation techniques, massage therapy, music therapy, and biofeedback enhance antiemetic effectiveness. Other benefits are that these interventions are relatively inexpensive and can be practiced by the individual.

  Behavioral interventions are also helpful in managing anticipatory nausea and vomiting.

- Acupuncture and acupressure may be helpful in reducing anticipatory nausea and vomiting.

Nutritional Modification for Nausea and Vomiting

- Change to a bland diet or foods that do not have offensive odor or spicy taste.
- Eat foods that are either cold or at room-temperature.

- Try clear liquids, carbonated beverages, and soda crackers.
- Avoid high-fat foods that can delay gastric emptying.
- Avoid favorite foods when nauseated.

Stomatitis and Mucositis

- *Stomatitis and mucositis* are general terms referring to inflammation and ulceration of the oral mucosa (Table 10-5) (Beck, 2004; Rubenstein, et al., 2004; McGuire, et al., 2004; McGuire, 2002).

TABLE 10-5

NCI Common Toxicity Grading Criteria for Stomatitis

Grade 0	Grade 1	Grade 2	Grade 3	Grade 4
None	Painless ulcers, erythema, or mild soreness	Painful erythema, edema, or ulcers but can eat	Painful erythema, edema, or ulcers and cannot eat	Requires parenteral or enteral support

- Oral mucosa is vulnerable to the effects of chemotherapy because the cells live for about 5 days and there is a rapid turnover of the epithelial lining every 7 to 14 days.
- Chemotherapy has a direct and indirect stomatoxic effect, and stomatitis is usually associated with chemotherapy.

- Fluorouracil is associated with a high degree of stomatitis.
- Other chemotherapy agents causing stomatitis include doxorubicin and methotrexate.
- Patients at higher risk for stomatitis

  Poor oral hygiene

  Presence of dental caries

  Chronic alcohol use
- Stomatitis is predictable and occurs within 2 to 5 days after treatment and can persist up to 14 days.
- Prevention strategies
    1. Primary goal is prevention of stomatitis.
    2. Implement a good oral hygiene program and maintain a good nutritional state.
    3. Agents used for oral care are cleansing agents (e.g., normal saline, hydrogen peroxide rinses) and lubricating agents (e.g., emollients).
- Management of mild to moderate stomatitis

  Assess oral cavity.

  Promote oral hygiene.

  Use mouth rinses.

  Change to a soft, high-calorie diet.

  Culture any suspicious oral lesions.

  Continue with cleansing agents and lubricating agents.

  Use topical anesthetics (e.g., benzocaine, Zilactin).

- Management of severe stomatitis

  Warm saline rinses

  Antifungal/antibacterial oral suspension

  Oxidizing agents

  Culture lesion and monitor for secondary oral infections

  Use topical/systemic analgesics

  Maintain hydration

Weight Gain

- Incidence of weight gain varies between 50% and 90%.
- Many women have weight gain greater than 10% of body weight.
- Mechanism of weight gain may be related to sarcopenic obesity.
- Gain may last up to 2 years posttreatment.
- Interventions

  Anticipatory guidance

  Documentation of weight

  Nutritional counseling

  Exercise (e.g., self-paced walking programs, fitness exercises)

Cancer-Related Fatigue (Nail, 2004)

- Guidelines for the management of cancer-related fatigue developed by the NCCN can be accessed online at www.nccn.org/professionals/physician_gls/PDF/fatigue.pdf.

- The reader is referred to Chapter 15 for further discussion of cancer-related fatigue (CRF).

- CRF is the persistent, subjective sense of tiredness related to cancer or cancer treatment that interferes with usual functioning (NCCN, 2004).

- CRF is the most frequently reported side effect of treatment.

- Screening for CRF

  1. Modeled on similar approach to pain assessment, using 0 to 10 scale, on which 0 is no fatigue and 10 is the most fatigue possible.

  2. Evaluate contributing factors to CRF including pain, distress, sleep disturbance, anemia, activity level, nutrition, and comorbidities (NCCN, 2004).

- Management of Mild CRF

  Provide preparatory education and discussion of common strategies to manage fatigue and its occurrence.

  Provide instructions about balance of energy conservation and appropriate exercise.

  Assist patients in prioritizing activities that differentiate essential from nonessential tasks.

  Promote a balance between sleep and rest. Patients who are fatigued may also experience accompanying symptom clusters of sleep disruption and mood disturbance.

  Evaluate the effectiveness of the interventions.

- Management of Moderate to Severe CRF

> *Consider nonpharmacologic approaches such as sleep therapy, restorative therapy, nutritional consultation, and psychosocial interventions.*
>
> *Consider pharmacologic management.*

- Exercise intervention for CRF

> *Research suggests that women receiving adjuvant chemotherapy benefit from either supervised or a self-administered walking exercise program.*

Arthralgia and Myalgia (Martin, 2004)

- Arthralgia is joint pain.
- Myalgia is diffuse muscle pain.
- Symptoms are dose related.

> *Paclitaxel at doses less than 170 mg/m^2 causes mild discomfort.*
>
> *Paclitaxel at doses greater than 200 mg/m^2 is associated with more severe discomfort and pain.*
>
> *Overlapping side effects of other chemotherapy include fatigue, malaise, decreased appetite, and lack of energy.*

- Symptom management:

> *Perform a careful assessment to identify risk factors.*
>
> *Inform patients as to what to expect, what can be prevented, and to whom to report side effects, and timeline of toxicity.*
>
> *Treatment approaches include antihistamines, corticosteroids, NSAIDs, opiates, warm bath, relaxation techniques, massage therapy.*

- Toxicity Criteria for Arthralgia and Myalgia listed on Table 10-6.

TABLE 10-6

NCI Common Toxicity Grading Criteria for Arthralgia and Myalgia

Grade 0	Grade 1	Grade 2	Grade 3	Grade 4
None	Mild pain; not interfering with function	Moderate pain; pain or analgesics interfering with function but not interfering with activities of daily living	Severe pain; pain or analgesics severely interfering with activities of daily living	Disabling

REFERENCES

Beck, S. (2004). Mucositis. In C. H. Yarbro, M. H. Frogge & M. Goodman (Eds.), *Cancer symptom management* (3rd ed., pp. 276–292). Sudbury, MA: Jones & Bartlett.

Geddie, P. I. (2004). Adjuvant chemotherapy. In K. H. Dow (Ed.), *Contemporary issues in breast cancer: A nursing persective* (2nd ed., pp. 134–145). Sudbury, MA: Jones & Bartlett.

Martin, V. (2004). Arthralgias and myalgias. In C. H. Yarbro, M. H. Frogge, & M. Goodman (Eds.), *Cancer symptom management* (3rd ed., pp. 17–28). Sudbury, MA: Jones & Bartlett.

McGuire, D. B. (2002). Mucosal tissue injury in cancer therapy. More than muscositis and mouthwash. *Cancer Practice, 10*(4), 179–191.

McGuire, D. B., Rubenstein, E. B., & Peterson, D. E. (2004). Evidence-based guidelines for managing mucositis. *Seminars in Oncology Nursing, 20*(1), 59–66.

Nail, L. (2004). Fatigue. In C. H. Yarbro, M. H. Frogge, & M. Goodman (Eds.), *Cancer symptom management* (3rd ed., pp. 47–60). Sudbury, MA: Jones & Bartlett.

National Comprehensive Cancer Network: http://www.nccn.org

Reeves, D. (2004). Alopecia. In C. H. Yarbro, M. H. Frogge, & M. Goodman (Eds.), *Cancer symptom management* (3rd ed., pp. 561–570). Sudbury, MA: Jones & Bartlett.

Rubenstein, E. B., Peterson, D. E., Schubert, M., Keefe, D., McGuire, D., Epstein, J., et al. (2004). Clinical practice guidelines for the prevention and treatment of cancer therapy-induced oral and gastrointestinal mucositis. *Cancer, 100*(9 Suppl), 2026–2046.

Wickham, R. (2004). Nausea and vomiting. In C. H. Yarbro, M. H. Frogge, & M. Goodman (Eds.), *Cancer symptom management* (3rd ed., pp. 187–214). Sudbury, MA: Jones & Bartlett.

Wujcik, D. (2004). Infection. In C. H. Yarbro, M. H. Frogge, & M. Goodman (Eds.), *Cancer symptom management* (3rd ed., pp. 252–275). Sudbury, MA: Jones & Bartlett.

CHAPTER ELEVEN

Hormonal Therapy

Use of Hormonal Therapy

- Beatson (1896) first recognized the dependence of breast tumors on estrogen for growth and proliferation.

- The roles of the estrogen receptor (ER) protein and the progesterone receptor (PR) protein in the proliferation of breast cancer tissue were identified in the 1960s.

- Estrogen, specifically estradiol, binds to ER sites on the nuclear cell membrane, stimulates gene transcription, and can result in cellular proliferation (Dienger, 2004).

- Thus, the risk of recurrence is a concern after treatment with surgery, radiation therapy, and/or chemotherapy.

- Hormonal therapy is the use of drugs that compete with estrogen for ER-binding sites.

- ER and PR status are used to evaluate prognosis and to predict response to hormonal therapy.
- About 80% of postmenopausal breast cancer is ER+ (positive) compared with about 50% of pre-menopausal breast cancer that is ER+.

Tamoxifen as Adjuvant Therapy

- Tamoxifen, a selective estrogen receptor modulator (SERM), was the first hormonal therapy used in the adjuvant treatment of breast cancer.
- Tamoxifen reduces the risk of recurrence by 47% and reduces the risk of death by 26% among women who took tamoxifen daily for 5 years (Early Breast Cancer Trialists' Collaborative Group, 1998a; 1998b).
- Tamoxifen has been evaluated extensively in clinical trials and has shown the efficacy of 5 years of treatment in preventing recurrence.
- Additional data support that continuation of tamoxifen beyond 5 years does not improve recurrence or disease free survival (Fisher, et al., 2001).
- Daily intake of tamoxifen 20 mg per day for 5 years has been the standard adjuvant hormone therapy for women with early-stage, hormone receptor positive breast cancer.
- SERMs have both estrogen antagonist and agonist effects.
- Tamoxifen acts as an estrogen antagonist by competing with estradiol for ER-binding sites and thus reducing cellular proliferation and tumor growth.

- Tamoxifen also reduces the production of insulin-derived growth factors and thus, decreases tumor growth.

- Tamoxifen acts as an estrogen agonist on other estrogen targets by increasing positive effects on blood lipid profiles and bone mineral density (Dienger, 2004; Osborne, 2004).

- Tamoxifen has been shown to reduce bone fractures in postmenopausal women who took tamoxifen for 5 years for the prevention of breast cancer (Fisher, et al., 1998).

- Tamoxifen is associated with a slight increased risk of endometrial cancer and venous thrombosis but the potential benefits of tamoxifen outweigh the risks for the majority of women.

- Hot flashes, vaginal discharge, and vaginal bleeding are bothersome with tamoxifen.

- Depression is an uncommon side effect, but when symptoms are severe, antidepressant medication, dose reduction, or even the discontinuation of tamoxifen has been recommended.

- Women with preexisting cataracts taking tamoxifen may have a slightly increased risk of posterior sub-capsular opacities but no vision-threatening ocular toxicity.

- Thrombolic and hematologic toxicities occur more frequently when tamoxifen is combined with chemotherapy.

- Severe thromboembolic events occur in less than 1% of patients.

- Endometrial and other cancers (e.g., liver cancer) are the most troublesome side effects of long-term tamoxifen.

- Endometrial cancer induced by tamoxifen is generally low grade, detected early, and treated with surgery.

- See Table 11-1 for the side effects of tamoxifen.

Aromatase Inhibitors

- Aromatase inhibitors are a class of hormonal therapy whose action is to inhibit estrogen synthesis by blocking the enzyme aromatase.

TABLE 11-1

Acute and Adverse Effects of Tamoxifen

Acute and Transient Effects	*Serious Adverse Effects*
Gastrointestinal upset	Thromboembolic events
Symptoms of estrogen withdrawal	Slightly elevated endometrial cancer risk
Hot flashes	Occular toxicity (retinopathy, cataracts)
Vaginal bleeding/discharge	
Menstrual irregularities in premenopausal women	
Irritability	
Depression	

- Aromatase is responsible for converting the adrenal androgens androstenedione and testosterone to estrone and estradiol in postmenopausal women.

- Aromatase inhibitors block estrogen synthesis and the availability of estrogen for binding at the ER sites.

- The aromatization reaction occurs in adipose tissue, muscle, and the liver.

- There are two classes of aromatase inhibitors (AI): steroidal and nonsteroidal inhibitors.

  Anastrozole and letrozole are nonsteroidal AIs and bind reversibly to the aromatase enzyme (Goss & Strasser, 2001; Ravdin, 2002).

  Exemestane is a steroidal AI that irreversibly inactivates the aromatase enzyme.

- Aromatase inhibitors were first introduced in the management of metastatic breast cancer and have since been approved as adjuvant hormonal therapy.

- Aromatase inhibitors, as single agents, have not been evaluated in premenopausal women and are not recommended outside of a clinical trial (Winer, et al., 2003).

Anastrozole

- Anastrozole is a selective, nonsteroidal aromatase inhibitor that was first used in the metastatic setting among postmenopausal women.

- Anastrozole 1 mg daily has low toxicity profile with **no** estrogen agonist effects.

- Because anastrozole has no agonist effects, the incidence of thromboembolic events and endometrial cancer are reduced (Dienger, 2004; Osborne, 2004).

- The efficacy of anastrozole in the adjuvant setting was evaluated in the ATAC trial (Arimidex, Tamoxifen, Alone or in Combination) (Buzdar, 2004).

- ATAC was designed to:
  1. evaluate the efficacy and safety of anastrozole compared to tamoxifen among postmenopausal ER+ women
  2. determine whether the combination of anastrozole and tamoxifen was superior to tamoxifen alone as adjuvant therapy in postmenopausal women

- The primary endpoint of ATAC was DFS (disease-free survival) and was defined as:

  Time to the earliest recurrence of local or distant recurrence

  New primary breast cancer

  Death from any cause

- The secondary endpoints were defined as:

  Time to recurrence

  Incidence of new contralateral primary breast tumor

- Eligibility criteria included postmenopausal women with ER+ or unknown operable invasive breast cancer who had completed primary surgery and chemotherapy.

- Randomization into three groups:

1. Anastrozole-alone group received anastrozole 1 mg plus tamoxifen placebo.

2. Tamoxifen-alone group received tamoxifen 20 mg plus anastrozole placebo.

3. Anstrozole + tamoxifen group received anastrozole 1 mg and tamoxifen 20 mg daily for 5 years.

-   A total of 9,366 postmenopausal women (mean age 64 years) were enrolled worldwide at the time the trial closed in 2000.

-   At a median follow-up of 33 months, the results showed (ATAC Trialists' Group, 2002).

    1. There were fewer number of primary contralateral breast cancers among women in the anastrozole group.

    2. No difference occurred in annual recurrence between the tamoxifen-alone or anastrozole-alone groups in the first year of follow-up.

    3. There was a difference favoring the anastrozole-alone group in the second and third year of follow-up.

    4. DFS was significantly longer for women in the anastrozole-alone group compared with the two other groups.

-   Hormonal receptor unknown status in subjects were later classified as hormone receptor negative and the results were reanalyzed to evaluate known hormone receptor status.

> *Women with ER+ tumors who were in the anastrozole-alone group had significantly larger DFS compared with the other groups.*
>
> *Recurrence rates were significantly higher among women with ER tumors.*

- These results led the researchers to conclude that:

  1. Anastrozole alone demonstrated better efficacy than the tamoxifen.

  2. The combination treatment with anastrozole + tamoxifen was equivalent to tamoxifen alone but slightly worse than anastrozole alone.

  3. Anastrozole was not more effective in women with ER disease.

- Side Effects and Quality of Life

  > *Hot flashes, fatigue, nausea, vomiting, headache, peripheral edema, constipation, bone pain, and back pain are the most common side effects.*
  >
  > *Table 11-2 lists the comparison of adverse effects among the three groups.*
  >
  > *Hot flashes, vaginal discharge, vaginal bleeding, ischemic cerebrovascular disease, deep venous thromboembolism, and endometrial cancers were significantly fewer in the anastrozole-alone group.*
  >
  > *In comparison, musculoskeletal effects and fractures were higher in the anastrozole-alone group.*
  >
  > *Fallowfield and associates (2004) also reported no differences in quality of life across the three groups during the first 2 years of treatment.*

TABLE 11-2
ATAC Trial: Comparison of Adverse Effects—
Percent of Incidence

	Anastrozole	Tamoxifen	Combination	p (A vs. T)
Hot flashes	34.3%	39.7%	40.1%	<0.0001
Musculoskeletal sx	27.8%	21.2%	22.1%	<0.0001*
Fatigue/tiredness	15.6%	15.1%	14.0%	0.5
Mood disturbances	15.5%	15.2%	15.6%	0.7
Nausea/vomiting	10.5%	10.2%	11.7%	0.7
Fractures	5.9%	3.7%	4.6%	<0.0001*
Vaginal bleeding	4.5%	8.2%	7.7%	<0.0001
Vaginal discharge	2.8%	11.4%	11.5%	<0.0001
Cataracts	3.5%	3.7%	3.4%	0.06
Thromboembolic	2.1%	3.5%	4.0%	0.0006
DVT/PE	1.0%	1.7%	2.0%	0.02
CVA	1.0%	2.1%	1.6%	0.0006
Endometrial ca	.1%	.5%	.3%	0.02

A = anastrozole; T = tamoxifen
* Significance in favor of tamoxifen

From "Anastrozole alone or in combination with tamoxifen versus
tamoxifen alone for adjuvant treatment of postmenopausal women
with early breast cancer: First results of the ATAC randomized trial"
by The ATAC Trialists' Group, 2002, *The Lancet, 359*, p 2136.
Adapted with permission.

- Although the ATAC results are promising, longer
  follow-up data beyond 33 months has been advo-
  cated to determine whether the improved response
  lasts for 5 years or more.

- The updated results of ATAC at a median of 47
  months of follow-up shows that anastrozole

continues to have better efficacy compared with tamoxifen including longer DFS and longer median time to recurrence (Buzdar, 2004).

- The Technology Assessment Workgroup of the American Society of Clinical Oncology (ASCO) reviewed the updated ATAC study results and found that there are no substantial differences in efficacy of toxicity associated and unanimously voted to support and maintain recommendations that were initially released in 2002 (Winer et al., 2003).

- ASCO 2002 recommendations are that the 5-year course of tamoxifen remain the standard adjuvant hormonal therapy for women with ER+ breast cancer.

- ASCO 2004 recommendations further suggested that:

  1. Anastrozole may be considered in post-menopausal women with ER+ tumors who have an absolute or relative contraindication to the use of tamoxifen.

  2. Contraindications may include women who are at increased risk of thromboembolic or cerebrovascular disease.

- Anastrozole has been approved by the FDA for the adjuvant treatment of postmenopausal breast cancer.

Letrozole

- Letrozole is an aromatase inhibitor that inhibits the peripheral conversion of androgens into estrogens and reduces the level of circulating estrogens by more than 95% in postmenopausal women (Smith & Dowsett, 2003).

- Letrozole is effective in the treatment of post-menopausal women with advanced breast cancer whose tumors are ER+.

- Goss and associates (2003) evaluated the safety and efficacy of letrozole after tamoxifen therapy in 5187 women with postmenopausal breast cancer in a double-blind, multicenter, international randomized trial.

- The primary endpoint was DFS.

- The planned interim analysis was done after 2.4 years of follow-up and showed that (Goss, et al., 2003):

    1. DFS was significantly higher in the letrozole group compared with the placebo group (P<.001).

    2. Results translate into a 2.2% difference in the rate of distant metastasis, ipsilateral recurrence, and new contralateral breast cancers.

    3. There were no differences in overall survival.

    4. Side effects of low-grade hot flashes, arthritis, arthralgia, and myalgia were more frequent in the letrozole group compared with placebo.

    5. Vaginal bleeding was less frequent in the letrozole group.

    6. Osteoporosis occurred in 5.8% of women in the letrozole group compared with 4.5% of women in the placebo group (P=.07).

- The results led to early termination of the study and the results were made public.
- Concerns raised with early termination included (Bryant & Wolmark, 2003; Burstein, 2003):
  1. None of the women received the planned 5 years of therapy with letrozole.
  2. There is limited data on the long-term effects of estrogen deprivation on bone density, cardiovascular health, and quality of life.
  3. The absolute benefits of leterozole therapy are limited to 2 to 3 years.
- Thus, women who are being considered for an aromatase inhibitor after tamoxifen therapy require additional instruction about the potential risks and benefits of treatment.
- The sequence and timing of tamoxifen and aromatase inhibitors for early-stage breast cancer is being evaluated in clinical trials.
- In October 2004, the FDA granted accelerated approval for letrozole for the extended adjuvant treatment of early-stage breast cancer in postmenopausal women who had received 5 years of adjuvant tamoxifen therapy.

Promising Directions for Adjuvant Hormonal Therapy

- Significant changes have occurred in the adjuvant use of hormonal therapy for breast cancer.

- Reduction in mortality is related to the use of adjuvant hormonal therapy.
- Some additional areas being addressed in clinical trials include (Osborne, 2004):
  1. The potential benefit of tamoxifen beyond 5 years of treatment in subgroups of women with breast cancer.
  2. The sequencing of tamoxifen with aromatase inhibitors.
  3. The role of aromatase inhibitors combined with ovarian ablation in premenopausal women.

REFERENCES

ATAC Trialists' Group. (2002). Anastrozole-alone or in combination with tamoxifen versus tamoxifen alone for adjuvant treatment of postmenopausal women with early breast cancer: First results of the ATAC randomized trial. *Lancet, 359,* 2131–2139.

Beatson, G. (1896). On the treatment of inoperable cases of carcinoma of the mamma: Suggestions for a new method of treatment, with illustrative cases. *Lancet, 2,* 104–107.

Bryant, J., & Wolmark, N. (2003). *Letrozole after tamoxifen for breast cancer—What is the price of success?* Retrieved October 13, 2003, from www.nejm.org

Burstein, H. (2003). *Beyond tamoxifen—Extending endocrine treatment for early stage breast cancer.* Retrieved October 13, 2003, from www.nejm.org

Buzdar, A. (2004). The ATAC (Arimidex, Tamoxifen, alone or in combination) trial update. *Clinical Breast Cancer, 5*, S6–S12.

Dienger, J. (2004). Hormonal therapy. In K. H. Dow (Ed.), *Contemporary issues in breast cancer: A nursing persective* (pp. 146–162). Sudbury, MA: Jones & Bartlett.

Early Breast Cancer Trialists' Collaborative Group. (1998a). Systemic treatment of early breast cancer by hormonal, cyto-toxic, or immune therapy: 133 randomised trials involving 31,000 recurrences and 24,000 deaths among 75,000 women. *Lancet, 339*, 71–85.

Early Breast Cancer Trialists' Collaborative Group. (1998b). Tamoxifen for early breast cancer: An overview of the random-ized trials. *Lancet, 351*(9114), 1451–1467.

Fallowfield, L., Cella, D., Cuzick, J., Francis, S., Locker, G., & Howell, A. (2004). Quality of life of postmenopausal women in the arimidex, tamoxifen, alone or in combination (ATAC) adju-vant breast cancer trial. *Journal of Clinical Oncology, 22*(21), 4261–4271.

Fisher, B., Costantino, J., Wickerham, D., & et al. (1998). Tamoxifen for prevention of breast cancer: Report of the National Surgical Adjuvant Breast and Bowel Project P-1 Study. *Journal of the National Cancer Institute, 16*, 1381–1388.

Fisher, B., Land, S., & Mamounas, E., et al. (2001). Prevention of invasive breast cancer in women with ductal carcinoma in situ. An update of the national surgical adjuvant bowel and breast project experience. *Seminars in Oncology, 28*(4), 400–418.

Goss, P., Ingle, J., Martino, S., Robert, N., Muss, H., Piccart, M., et al. (2003). A randomized trial of letrozole in postmenopausal women after five years of tamoxifen therapy for early-stage breast cancer. *The New England Journal of Medicine, 349*, 1793–1802.

Goss, P., & Strasser, K. (2001). Aromatase inhibitors in the treatment and prevention of breast cancer. *Journal of Clinical Oncology, 19*, 881–894.

Osborne, C. K. (2004). Adjuvant endocrine therapy. In J. R. Harris, M. E. Lippman, M. Morrow, & C. K. Osborne (Eds.), *Diseases of the breast* (3rd ed., pp. 865–892). Philadelphia: Lippincott Williams & Wilkins.

Ravdin, P. (2002). Aromatase inhibitors for the endocrine adjuvant treatment of breast cancer. *Lancet, 359*, 2126–2127.

Smith, I. E., & Dowsett, M. (2003). Aromatase inhibitors in breast cancer. *New England Journal of Medicine, 348*(24), 2431–2442.

Winer, P., Hudis, C., Burstein, H. J., Bryant, J., Chlebowski, R. T., Ingle, J., et al. (2003). American Society of Clinical Oncology Technology assessment on the use of aromatase inhibitors as adjuvant therapy for postmenopausal women with hormone receptor-positive breas cancer: Status Report 2004. *Journal of Clinical Oncology, 23*(3): 619–629. Epub 2004 Nov. 15.

PART III

Management of Recurrent Breast Cancer

CHAPTER TWELVE

Local Management of Recurrent Disease

Introduction

- *Local recurrence* is the reappearance of cancer in the ipsilateral breast, chest wall, or skin overlying the chest wall after initial treatment.

- *Regional recurrence* is the appearance of tumor involving the ipsilateral axillary lymph nodes, supraclavicular lymph nodes, infraclavicular lymph nodes, and internal mammary lymph nodes.

- *Distant recurrence* (also known as *metastasis*) is the reappearance of cancer in bone or organs.

- Local recurrence may occur after either mastectomy or breast-conserving surgery (BCS) and radiation therapy (XRT).

- In general, treatment for recurrence after mastectomy is surgical resection of recurrence and radiation therapy. Treatment for recurrence after BCS and XRT is total mastectomy.

- After local treatment is complete, patients are considered candidates for systemic chemotherapy or hormonal therapy.

Local Recurrence After Mastectomy (Recht, et al., 2000)

- Local recurrence often presents as one or more asymptomatic nodules in or under the skin of the chest wall.

- Nodules may be found in or near the mastectomy scar or skin graft and after myocutaneous flap reconstruction.

- Recurrence may look like an erythematous, pruritic skin rash.

- Eighty percent to 90% of local recurrences occur within 5 years after mastectomy.

- Twenty-five percent to 33% of patients with local or regional recurrence have distant metastasis before local recurrence is found.

- About 25% of patients develop simultaneous local and distant metastasis within a few months after local recurrence.

- Unfortunately, nearly all patients with local recurrence after mastectomy develop distant metastasis.

- Patients with local recurrence.

Local Management of Recurrence After Mastectomy

- XRT is generally delivered to the chest wall and supraclavicular nodes.

  With a higher dose of radiation to a large chest wall field and nodal irradiation, the higher is the likelihood of local control.

  Recurrence in a mastectomy scar may be more difficult to control, compared with other chest wall recurrence.

  Patients who have local failure after mastectomy and reconstruction have control rates and outcomes similar to other patients without reconstruction.

  Radiation to the internal mammary nodes requires a larger volume of lung and heart (for left-sided lesions) in the treatment field, which may increase patient morbidity, particularly after prior doxorubicin-based adjuvant therapy.

  Axillary radiation is not generally done unless there is clinical involvement or minimal dissection.

- Radiation treatment consists of either photon radiation or mixed photon-electron beam radiation (Recht, et al., 2000)

  45 to 50 Gy (Gy = Gray; measure of radiation dose), using photons delivered in 1.8- to 2.0-Gy fractions five times a week to chest wall

  10- to 20-Gy boost with photons or electrons to areas of gross disease and biopsy

  Total radiation dose is generally 60 Gy

- Side effects and complications

  Acute side effects include a brisk skin redness and possible desquamation.

  Complications include telangiectasia and mild subcutaneous fibrosis.

  Serious complications, such as radiation pneumonitis, soft-tissue necrosis, bone necrosis, and neuropathy, are rare.

  Concurrent administration of chemotherapy may increase the risk of pneumonitis, pericarditis, and brachial plexopathy.

Local Management of Recurrence After Breast-Conserving Surgery and Radiation Therapy (BCS+XRT) (Solin, et al., 2004)

- About 50% of local recurrence after BCS and XRT are detected by mammography.

- Physical and radiologic characteristics of recurrent tumors are similar to those of initial tumors.

- Physical examination shows mild thickening without a mass; in some patients, recurrence may produce only mild thickening or retraction at the biopsy site.

- Prognosis after recurrence in BCS+XRT is better than local recurrence after mastectomy.

- Treatment with salvage mastectomy is the standard therapy. Mastectomy has a 5-year, relapse-free survival rate of about 60% to 75%.

- Postoperative complications include delayed wound healing and infection.
- Patients desiring immediate reconstruction may have a higher risk of delayed wound healing and a variable cosmetic result because of prior XRT.

Common Sites of Distant Metastasis

- Breast cancer can metastasize to other areas in the body.
- One of the most frequent sites of metastasis is to the bone. Bone metastasis is considered an oncologic emergency in situations when there may be an impending fracture.
- Two additional sites of distant metastasis that are considered oncologic emergencies are to the spinal cord, causing compression and brain metastasis, causing seizures.

Bone Metastases (Theriault, 2000)

- Most frequent site of metastasis, with about 90% of patients with metastatic disease having bone metastases.
- Lesions may be osteolytic, osteoblastic, mixed osteolytic-osteoblastic, and osteoporotic, leading to pathologic fractures of weight-bearing bones.
- Bone metastases occur in trabecular bone and cortical bones.

- Most common involved sites include pelvis, lumbar spine, thoracic spine, ribs, long bones, skull, and cervical spine.

- Bone metastasis is associated with bone loss and excess excretion of calcium.

- Symptoms of pain and disability cause major problems in quality of life.

- Work-up for bone metastases:

  Physical examination, bone scan, and plain films are conducted.

  Computed tomography (CT) and MRI also may be used in the evaluation.

Management of Bone Metastasis: Radiation Therapy and Systemic Radionuclide Therapy

- Radiation therapy has been used for pain relief and prevention of impending pathologic fracture.

- Hemibody radiation has been used when there are multiple bony lesions in the spine.

- The side effects of radiation therapy for bone metastasis are skin erythema in the treatment field and mild to moderate fatigue.

- Strontium-89 and samarium-153 are radionucles that may be given by intravenous injection for relief of bone pain.

  These agents are taken up at sites of active bone mineral turnover and are most often used in patients with diffuse bony metastasis.

> *These agents are FDA approved for adult and pediatric relief of metastatic bone pain.*
>
> *Hematologic toxicity is dose-limiting toxicity.*

- Pain management for bone metastasis

> *Patients require an effective pain control regimen during XRT.*
>
> *Combination of opioid and nonopioid (NSAID) helps relieve pain during XRT.*

Management of Bone Metastasis: Bisphosphonates

- Bisphosphonates are analogues of pyrophosphate and have been shown to inhibit osteoclast-mediated bone destruction.

- Bisphosphonates bind at sites of active bone remodeling.

- The degree by which bisphosphonates inhibit osteoclast function varies based on structure with amino-containing agents (e.g., risedronate, pamidronate, alendronate, and zoledronate) being more potent than the nonamino-containing agents (e.g., clodronate, etidronate).

- The American Society of Clinical Oncology (ASCO) update on the role of bisphosphonates and bone health issues in women with breast cancer can be accessed online at http://asco.org/ac/1,1003,_12-002032-00_18-0031101,00.asp.

Bisphosphonates reduce skeletal complications, such as pathologic fracture, surgery for fracture or impending fracture, XRT, spinal cord compression, and hypercalcemia (Hillner, et al., 2003).

Bisphosphonates provide a supportive but no life-prolonging benefit in patients with bone metastases.

The ASCO guidelines recommend intravenous pamidronate 90 mg delivered over 2 hours or zoledronic acid 4 mg over 15 minutes every 3 to 4 weeks. Patients' creatinine must be monitored before each dose of either drug.

Epidural Spinal Cord Compression (Wen, et al., 2004; Bucholtz, 1999)

- Epidural spinal cord compression (ESCC) is considered an oncologic emergency.

- Predictors of spinal cord compression include known bone metastases to the spine of at least 2 years, metastatic disease at initial diagnosis, and weakness (Lu, et al., 1998).

- Spinal cord damage is due to direct compression of the spinal cord by the tumor.

- Breast cancer accounts for 7% to 32% of all cases of spinal cord compression.

- Signs and symptoms

    Pain is the most common initial symptom and precedes other symptoms by several weeks.

> *Pain may be local, radicular, and referred, and the type of pain is further described in Table 12-1.*
>
> *Pain worsens when patients are lying down and when patients use stretch maneuvers such as neck flexion.*
>
> *Myelopathy symptoms such as limb weakness, numbness, paresthesias, and sphincter disturbance may occur.*
>
> *Prognosis with spinal cord compression is related to clinical deficits at the time of presentation.*

- If left untreated, ESCC complications include paraplegia or quadriplegia.
- Work-up includes plain spine films, radionuclide bone scan, CT and MRI of the spine.

TABLE 12-1

Types of Pain Related to Spinal Cord Compression

Type of Pain	Description of Pain
Local	Described as a constant ache
	Occurs in nearly all patients
Radicular	Described as a shooting pain
	Caused by involvement of nerve roots by the tumor
	More common in cervical and lumbosacral lesions
Referred	Occurs at a site distant from the lesion
	Pain does not radiate
	Lesions in the lower thoracic and lumbar spine may be referred to iliac crests or sacroiliac joints
	Lesions in low cervical and high thoracic regions may be referred to interscapular region or shoulders

Management of ESCC

- Corticosteroids

  Routinely used to reduce pain and stabilize neurologic deficits

  Usually, a larger bolus dose of dexamethasone, followed by a tapering dose over several weeks while patient receives definitive therapy.

- Radiation therapy

  Emergency treatment with XRT should be started on an urgent basis.

  Recommended first-line treatment, using a dose up to 30 Gy delivered in 3-Gy fractions to the targeted area in spine.

  General skin-care measures are used during XRT.

  XRT for SCC may result in mild to moderate local side effects, depending on the bodily structures in the path of the radiation beam.

  XRT to the spine may cause dysphagia.

  1. Nutritional measures, such as increasing liquids and instituting a soft diet

  2. Local anesthetic for pain

- Decompressive laminectomy

  May be used in selected situations in which the patient's disease progresses or relapses with XRT

  Has had limited effectiveness compared with radiation therapy

- Chemotherapy and hormonal therapy have a very limited role in the treatment of ESCC.

Brain Metastases (Ramakrishna, et al., 2004; Fokstuen, et al, 2000; Ogura, et al., 2003; Wen & Shafman, 2000; Lin, et al., 2004)

- Brain metastases is the most common neurologic complication in breast cancer, occurring in about 14–20% of patients (Ramakrishna, et al., 2004).

- The majority of patients are treated with palliative external beam whole-brain XRT, with relief of symptoms occurring in about 45% of patients.

- Median time from diagnosis to CNS metastases is about 33 months, with median survival after treatment of about 4 months (Fokstuen, et al., 2000).

- Patients with singular brain metastasis with postoperative radiation have better survival, compared with patients with multiple brain metastases and meningeal spread (Ogura, et al., 2003; Wen & Shafman, 2000).

- Hematogenous spread is the most common mechanism of brain metastases.

- Brain metastases are more likely to occur in premenopausal women with aggressive and disseminated disease (Lin, et al., 2004).

- Development of brain metastases is delayed in patients who received adjuvant chemotherapy or hormonal therapy, but overall survival is not affected.

- Trastuzumab does not cross the blood brain barrier and the rate of CNS metastases in patients who receive this agent has been a recent concern. Lai and colleagues (2004) conducted a retrospective cohort study of 343 patients and found no evidence of an association between trastuzumab and an increased risk of CNS metastasis.

- Signs and symptoms vary, with the majority of patients presenting with progressive neurologic deficits, cognitive dysfunction, and seizure.

    Clinical manifestations include headache, altered mental status, hemiparesis, papilledema, and ataxia.

    Cognitive dysfunction includes memory problems and mood or personality changes.

- Work-up

    CT scan detects the majority of brain metastases.

    Contrast-enhanced MRI is more sensitive than CT.

- Treatment of brain metastasis includes radiation therapy, stereotactic radiosurgery, and surgery.

- Chemotherapy and hormonal therapy have a limited role in the palliative treatment of brain metastasis.

Management of Brain Metastases

- Corticosteroids with dexamethasone are routinely used to reduce symptomatic edema.

    Patients have symptomatic relief within a few days after starting treatment.

    Side effects of corticosteroids include weight gain, myopathy, fluid retention, hyperglycemia, insomnia, gastritis, and immunosuppression.

- Anticonvulsant therapy in patients presenting with seizures

  Routine anticonvulsant therapy in patients who have not experienced seizure is not indicated.

  The side effect of drug rashes is not uncommon.

- Treatment is delivered on an emergency basis.

- Goals of definitive treatment are symptomatic relief of symptoms and improvement of local control of disease.

- XRT to whole brain on an emergency basis and surgery are the major treatments for brain metastases.

Radiation Therapy for Brain Metastasis

- XRT is the standard treatment of brain metastases and is also effective in palliating neurologic symptoms.

- Up to 90% high response with radiation to decrease neurologic symptoms.

- Whole-brain radiation-dose fractionation schedules vary from 20 Gy in 5 fractions to 40 Gy in 20 fractions.

- In general, patients who are treated in the shortest amount of time with larger radiation treatment fractions tend to respond more quickly.

- Duration of response is equivalent with fractionation schedules.

- Late complications of XRT are rare but may include leukoencephalopathy, neurocognitive deterioration, and dementia.

- Stereotactic radiosurgery delivers a high single dose of radiation to a specific treatment volume. It has been used as an alternative to surgery or whole-brain radiation therapy. Stereotactic radiosurgery uses high-energy X-rays from a linear accelerator or with gamma rays from a gamma knife.
- Side effects of XRT to the whole brain (Bucholtz, 1997):
  1. Complete but temporary hair loss within a few weeks of start of XRT, with hair regrowth after treatment ends
  2. Scalp dryness and itchiness
  3. Skin erythema (especially in forehead and periauricular areas)
  4. Fatigue
  5. Potential for a transient increase in neurologic symptoms at start of XRT
- Patient safety at home
  1. Assess degree of cognitive impairment and need for home safety.
  2. Monitor taper of steroids at the end of the treatment course.
  3. Provide emotional support to patient and family.

Surgery for Brain Metastases
- Surgery is used for treatment of single brain metastases that may be surgically resectable, which may be followed by stereotactic radiosurgery.

- Surgery may be used for treatment of multiple brain metastases with large symptomatic lesions, followed by whole-brain radiation.

- There is improved safety of surgery for brain metastasis as a result of advances in neurosurgery, neuroanesthesia, and use of computer assisted stereotactic techniques.

REFERENCES

Bucholtz, J. (1997). Central nervous system tumors. In K. H. Dow, J. D. Bucholtz, R. Iwamoto, V. Fieler, & L. Hilderly (Eds.), *Nursing care in radiation oncology* (2nd ed., pp. 136–151). Philadelphia: WB Saunders.

Bucholtz, J. D. (1999). Metastatic epidural spinal cord compression. *Seminars in Oncology Nursing, 15*(3), 150–159.

Fokstuen, T., Wilking, N., Rutqvist, L. E., Wolke, J., Liedberg, A., Signomklao, T., et al. (2000). Radiation therapy in the management of brain metastases from breast cancer. *Breast Cancer Research and Treatment, 62*(3), 211–216.

Hillner, B. E., Ingle, J. N., Chlebowski, R. T., Gralow, J., Yee, G. C., Janjan, N. A., et al. (2003). American Society of Clinical Oncology 2003 update on the role of bisphosphonates and bone health issues in women with breast cancer. *Journal of Clinical Oncology, 21*(21), 4042–4057.

Lai, R., Dang, C. T., Malkin, M. G., & Abrey, L. E. (2004). The risk of central nervous system metastases after trastuzumab therapy in patients with breast carcinoma. *Cancer, 101*(4), 810–816.

Lin, N. U., Bellon, J. R., & Winer, E. P. (2004). CNS metastases in breast cancer. *Journal of Clinical Oncology, 22*(17), 3608–3617.

Lu, C., Stomper, P., Drislane, F., et al. (1998). Suspected spinal cord compression in breast cancer patients: A multidisciplinary risk assessment. *Breast Cancer Research & Treatment, 51*(2), 121–131.

Ogura, M., Mitsumori, M., Okumura, S., Yamauchi, C., Kawamura, S., Oya, N., et al. (2003). Radiation therapy for brain metastases from breast cancer. *Breast Cancer, 10*(4), 349–355.

Ramakrishna, N., Galper, S., & Wen, P. Y. (2004). Brain metastases. In J. R. Harris, M. Lippman, M. Morrow, & C. K. Osborne (Eds.), *Diseases of the breast* (3rd ed., pp. 1205–1218). Philadelphia: Lippincott Williams & Wilkins.

Recht, A., Come, S., Troyan, S., & Sadowsky, N. (2000). Local-regional recurrence after mastectomy or breast-conserving therapy. In J. R. Harris, M. Lippman, M. Morrow, & C. K. Osborne (Eds.), *Diseases of the breast* (2nd ed., pp. 731–748). Philadelphia: Lippincott Williams & Wilkins.

Solin, L. J., Harris, E. R., Orel, S. G., & Glick, J. H. (2004). Local-regional recurrence after breast conservation treatment or mastectomy. In J. R. Harris, M. Lippman, M. Morrow, & C. K. Osborne (Eds.), *Diseases of the breast* (3rd ed., pp. 1067–1087). Philadelphia: Lippincott Williams & Wilkins.

Theriault, R. (2000). Medical treatment of bone metastases. In J. R. Harris, M. Lippman, M. Morrow, & C. K. Osborne (Eds.), *Diseases of the breast* (2nd ed., pp. 921–929). Philadelphia: Lippincott Williams & Wilkins.

Wen, P. Y., & Shafman, T. (2000). Brain metastasis. In J. R. Harris, M. Lippman, M. Morrow, & C. K. Osborne (Eds.), *Diseases of the breast* (2nd ed., pp. 841–853). Philadelphia: Lippincott Williams & Wilkins.

Wen, P. Y., McColl, C. D., & Freilich, R. J. (2004). Epidural metastases. In J. R. Harris, M. Lippman, M. Morrow, & C. K. Osborne (Eds.), *Diseases of the breast* (3rd ed., pp. 1219–1230). Philadelphia: Lippincott Williams & Wilkins.

CHAPTER THIRTEEN

Chemotherapy and Targeted Therapy in Recurrent Disease

Introduction and Overview (Ellis, et al., 2003)

- The goal of treatment is aimed at the management of symptoms, maintenance of or improvement in the quality of life, and possibly increased survival. Treatment is not curative. Assessment of risk and benefit of treatment modalities on quality of life must be reviewed prior to the start of treatment (Ellis, et al., 2003).

  Some patients are willing to accept a high degree of toxicity for even small survival benefits.

  Other patients prefer minimal toxicity with some degree of symptom palliation.

- Must establish the diagnosis of metastatic disease

  Histologic diagnosis of suspicious lesions is needed to select therapy

- Favorable prognostic indicators

  1. Longer time interval between primary diagnosis and relapse of more than 5 years after treatment is a favorable prognostic indicator

  2. Number and sites of metastatic disease with isolated sites of recurrence in the bone-versus-organ involvement

- Visceral involvement is a poor prognostic indicator in metastasis.

- There are two classes of therapeutic options: local or systemic. See Chapter 12 for a further discussion of local treatment of recurrence.

  1. Systemic therapy includes endocrine therapy, chemotherapy, or targeted therapy. See Chapter 14 for a further discussion of systemic treatment with endocrine therapy.

  2. Local therapy

- The selection of local, systemic therapy, targeted therapy, or combination of therapies is individualized.

Indications for Chemotherapy

- Patients with the following characteristics are considered candidates for chemotherapy:

1. Patients with negative ER and PR
2. Patients having a short disease-free interval
3. Patients with multiple metastatic sites and/or rapidly progressing visceral disease
4. Patients whose disease is nonresponsive to endocrine therapy

- Patients who are chemotherapy naïve have a higher likelihood of benefiting from chemotherapy.
- Patients who may have a poor response to chemotherapy include those with:

  Progression of disease while on prior chemotherapy

  Recurrence within 12 months after completing adjuvant chemotherapy

  Poor performance status

Chemotherapy in Recurrent Breast Cancer (Ellis, et al., 2003)

- Guidelines for the treatment of recurrent breast cancer developed by the National Comprehensive Cancer Network (NCCN) can be accessed online at www.nccn.org/professionals/physician_gls/PDF/breast.pdf.
- The selection of the type of chemotherapy and targeted therapy as either monotherapy or sequential therapy is based on several patient factors.
- First-line chemotherapy

First-line chemotherapy includes sequential single agents or combination chemotherapy.

1. *Single agents include anthracyclines, taxanes, capecitabine, vinorelbine, and gemcitabine (Miles, et al., 2004; O'Shaughnessy, et al., 2004; Miller, et al., 2001; Seidman, 2001; Gradishar, 2001; Hortobagyi, 2001).*

2. *Combination regimens include fluorouracil, doxorubicine, and cyclophosphamide (FAC/CAF); cyclophosphamide, epirubicin, and fluorouracil (CEF); doxorubicin and cyclophosphamide (AC); cyclophosphamide, methotrexate, and fluorouracil (CMF); and docetaxel, capecitabine (Nabholtz, et al., 2001; Pagani, et al., 2000).*

*   In addition to the chemotherapy drugs identified in Chapter 9, the agents in Table 13-1 are used in the treatment of metastatic disease.

Targeted Therapy (Slamon, et al., 2001; Bell, et al., 2004; Jones & Leyland-Jones, 2004)

*   Amplification and overexpression of protooncogene HER2 or c-erb-b^2 is used to select patients for targeted trastuzumab therapy in metastatic disease (Slamon, 2001; Bell, 2004).

    C-erb-b^2 encodes a 185 kD transmembrane glycoprotein with tyrosine kinase activity that functions as a growth factor receptor.

TABLE 13-1

Chemotherapy Used in Metastatic Breast Cancer

Capecitabine (Xeloda)

Mechanism of action	Orally administered prodrug that converts to fluorouracil intracellularly
Indications/Use	Metastatic breast cancer resistant to anthracyclines and paclitaxel or cancer resistant to paclitaxel for whom further anthracycline therapy is not indicated
Special precautions	Diarrhea may be more severe in elderly patients
Toxicity	Diarrhea may be severe
	Hand and foot syndrome
	Dermatitis
	Grade 3–4 hematologic toxicity (neutropenia and thrombocytopenia)
	Nausea and vomiting: common
	Fatigue
	Anorexia and abdominal pain less common

Gemcitabine (Gemzar, difluorodeoxycitidine)

Mechanism of action	Antimetabolite
	Nucleoside analog inhibits ribonucleotide reductase and competes with deoxycytidine triphosphate for incorporation into DNA
Special precautions	Irritant
	Administration: IV over 30 minutes up to 4 hours diluted in 100–200 cc of saline
	If >2,500 mg/m^2, dilute in 1,000 ml and infuse over 4 hours or longer
	Toxicity increased with longer infusion time

(*continues*)

TABLE 13-1 *(continued)*
Chemotherapy Used in Metastatic Breast Cancer

Gemcitabine (Gemzar, difluorodeoxycitidine) (continued)

Toxicity	Myelosuppression: common; dose limiting
	Nausea and vomiting: common, not severe
	Diarrhea: occasional
	Constipation
	Rash, fever, flu-like symptoms with first dose
	Alopecia
	Increase in liver function tests

Vinorelbine (Navelbine)

Mechanism of action	Semisynthetic vinca alkaloid
	Inhibits tubulin polymerization, inhibits mitosis
Indications/Use	Metastatic breast cancer
Special precautions	Vesicant
Toxicity	Myelosuppression: dose limiting; nadir 7–10 days
	Nausea and vomiting: common; mild to moderate
	Neurotoxicity: less common than seen with vincristine
	Constipation, occasional paresthesia, tumor and jaw pain
	Alopecia: occasional
	Allergic reaction: chest pain, dyspnea, wheezing during administration; may premedicate with corticosteroids
	Be alert for chest pain in patients with tumor in chest or history of cardiovascular disease

Source: Perry, et al., 1999; Skeel, 1999; Wilkes, et al., 2000

> *Amplified or overexpressed HER2/neu occurs in 25% to 30% of human breast cancer and is associated with rapid proliferation, growth, and metastasis.*
>
> *Trastuzumab is an anti-HER2 monoclonal antibody indicated in patients with metastatic breast cancer with overexpression of HER2, for first-line therapy with paclitaxel.*
>
> *The addition of trastuzumab to first-line chemotherapy in metastatic breast cancer is associated with a higher rate and duration of response and longer survival (Hortobagyi, 2001; Jones & Leyland, 2004).*
>
> *Trastuzumab can result in the development of ventricular dysfunction and congestive heart failure in patients who have received prior doxorubicin-containing regimens or in combination with doxorubicin. Left ventricular function is evaluated in patients prior to and during treatment with trastuzumab.*
>
> *See Table 13-2.*

- Patients with HER2 (erb-B^2) overexpression may benefit from the use of trastuzumab as a single agent or in combination with chemotherapeutic agents.

- Chemotherapy regimens used in combination with trastuzumab include paclitaxel + carboplatin, docetaxel + carboplatin, and vinorelbine.

- Trastuzumab in combination with doxorubicin/cyclophosphamide has about a 27% frequency of significant cardiac dysfunction. Thus, the combination has not been recommended in clinical practice outside of a clinical trial based on NCCN guidelines.

TABLE 13-2
Targeted Therapy in Metastatic Breast Cancer

Trastuzumab (Herceptin)

Mechanism of action	Recombinant humanized monoclonal anti-HER2 antibody
	Targets extracellular domain of HER2 growth factor receptor
	Inhibits signal transduction and cell proliferation
Indications/Use	Overexpression/amplification of HER2/neu (c-erbB-2) metastatic breast cancer
Special precautions	During first infusion, mild to moderate chills and fever that usually abate with subsequent treatment
	Cardiotoxicity is a complication and may occur in patients previously treated with anthracyclines.
Toxicity	Nausea and vomiting, pain are infrequent side effects.
	Other side effects include increased anemia, leukopenia, diarrhea, and infection.

Symptom Management

- Side effects are similar to adjuvant chemotherapy and include neutropenia, nausea and vomiting, weight gain, alopecia, fatigue, arthralgias, and myalgias.

- In addition, there are side effects related to capecitabine and include hand and foot syndrome and diarrhea (Mrozek-Orlowski, et al., 1999; Wagstaff, et al., 2003).

1. Hand and foot syndrome (HFS)

    •   Dose: limiting toxicity that usually appears during the first cycle of capecitabine but can occur anytime during treatment.

    •   In early mild stages, HFS is a tingling sensation accompanied by mild erythema, painless swelling, tenderness, rash, or dry and itchy skin on the palms of the hand and soles of the feet.

    •   Patients must stop taking the medication and wait until HFS resolves before restarting the medication.

    •   Emollients and creams containing lanolin and vitamin B are helpful.

    •   HFS can progress to painful erythema, swelling of the hands and feet, and blistering and severe pain. When severe side effects occur, patients must discontinue therapy until the toxicity resolves. Dose modification may be necessary when patients restart the medication.

2. Diarrhea is thought to be a result from antiproliferative activity on epithelial cells in the GI mucosa. Treatment of diarrhea is with loperamide and diet modification.

    •   Drug interactions occur with antacids that contain magnesium and aluminum-hydroxides that can affect the absorption of capecitabine.

- Bleeding levels are also affected when patients are on warfarin or phenytoin in combination with capecitabine.

Nursing Management in Recurrent Breast Cancer (Dow, 2004)

- The care of patients with recurrent breast cancer is complex. Nursing management focuses on the control of side effects, support and education, and helping the patient and family plan to maintain level of functioning with the least amount of disruption.

- The dilemmas facing women with advanced disease include but are not limited to:
  1. Restart course of treatment
  2. Manage side effects
  3. Face major changes in role responsibilities at home and at work
  4. Face the difficulties of a shortened life expectancy
  5. Manage an uncertain future

- Provide emotional support and strengthen coping abilities.
  1. Help spouses, significant others, children, and other family members understand issues in advanced breast cancer.
  2. Refer patient and family to supportive networks, groups, and social workers.

REFERENCES

Bell, R., Verma, S., Untch, M., Cameron, D., & Smith, I. (2004). Maximizing clinical benefit with trastuzumab. *Seminars in Oncology, 31*(5 Suppl 10), 35–44.

Dow, K. H. (2004). Targeted therapy and treatment of recurrent and metastatic breast cancer. In K. H. Dow (Ed.), *Contemporary issues in breast cancer: A nursing persective* (2nd ed., pp. 163–174). Sudbury, MA: Jones & Bartlett.

Ellis, M., Hayes, D., & Lippman, M. (2003). Treatment of metastatic breast cancer. In J. R. Harris, M. Lippman, M. Morrow, & C. K. Osborne (Eds.), *Diseases of the breast* (2nd ed., pp. 749–797). Philadelphia: Lippincott Williams & Wilkins.

Gradishar, W. J. (2001). Clinical status of capecitabine in the treatment of breast cancer. *Oncology (Huntington), 15*(1 Suppl 2), 69–71.

Hortobagyi, G. N. (2001). Treatment of advanced breast cancer with gemcitabine and vinorelbine. *Oncology (Huntington), 15*(2 Suppl 3), 15–17.

Jones, A. L., & Leyland-Jones, B. (2004). Optimizing treatment of HER2-positive metastatic breast cancer. *Seminars in Oncology, 31*(5 Suppl 10), 29–34.

Miles, D., Vukelja, S., Moiseyenko, V., Cervantes, G., Mauriac, L., Hazel, G. V., et al. (2004). Survival benefit with capecitabine/docetaxel versus docetaxel alone: Analysis of therapy in a randomized phase III trial. *Clinical Breast Cancer, 5*(4), 273–278.

Miller, K. D., Sisk, J., Ansari, R., Gize, G., Nattam, S., Pennington, K., et al. (2001). Gemcitabine, paclitaxel, and trastuzumab in metastatic breast cancer. *Oncology, 15*(2 Suppl 3), 38–40.

Mrozek-Orlowski, M. E., Frye, D. K., & Sanborn, H. M. (1999). Capecitabine: Nursing implications of a new oral chemotherapeutic agent. *Oncology Nursing Forum, 26*(4), 753–762.

Nabholtz, J. M., Mackey, J. R., Smylie, M., Paterson, A., Noel, D. R., Al-Tweigeri, T., et al. (2001). Phase II study of docetaxel, doxorubicin, and cyclophosphamide as first-line chemotherapy for metastatic breast cancer. *J Clin Oncol, 19*(2), 314–321.

O'Shaughnessy, J. A., Vukelja, S., Marsland, T., Kimmel, G., Ratnam, S., & Pippen, J. E. (2004). Phase II study of trastuzumab plus gemcitabine in chemotherapy-pretreated patients with metastatic breast cancer. *Clinical Breast Cancer, 5*(2), 142–147.

Pagani, O., Sessa, C., Nole, F., Crivellari, D., Lombardi, D., Thurlimann, B., et al. (2000). Epidoxorubicin and docetaxel as first-line chemotherapy in patients with advanced breast cancer: a multicentric phase I-II study. *Annals of Oncology, 11*(8), 985–991.

Perry, M. C., Anderson, C., Dorr, V., & Wilkes, J. (1999). *Companion handbook to the chemotherapy sourcebook.* Philadelphia: Lippincott Williams & Wilkins.

Seidman, A. D. (2001). The evolving role of gemcitabine in the management of breast cancer. *Oncology, 60*(3), 189–198.

Skeel, R. (1999). *Handbook of cancer chemotherapy* (5th ed.). Philadelphia: Lippincott Williams & Wilkins.

Slamon, D. J., Leyland-Jones, B., Shak, S., & et al. (2001). Use of chemotherapy plus a monoclonal antibody against HER2 for metastatic breast cancer that overexpresses HER2. *New England Journal of Medicine, 344*, 783–792.

Wagstaff, A. J., Ibbotson, T., & Goa, K. L. (2003). Capecitabine: A review of its pharmacology and therapeutic efficacy in the management of advanced breast cancer. *Drugs, 63*(2), 217–236.

Wilkes, G., Ingwersen, K., & Barton-Burke, M. (2000). *2000 oncology nursing drug handbook.* Sudbury, MA: Jones & Bartlett.

CHAPTER FOURTEEN

Endocrine Therapy in Recurrent Disease

Background (Ellis, et al., 2004)

- Beatson was the first to observe and document the regression of breast cancer after oophorectomy in 1896 and published the first paper on estrogen-dependent breast cancer.

- Ablative procedures to remove ovaries and endocrine organs resulted in oophorectomy, adrenalectomy, and hypophysectomy, but there was high morbidity associated with surgery.

- In the 1960s, pharmacologic approaches replaced ablative procedures with estrogens such as diethylstilbestrol (DES) and conjugated estrogens. However, major side effects, such as nausea, vomiting, uterine bleeding, edema, thrombolytic event, and congestive heart failure, limited the use of these early pharmacologic agents. Newer endocrine therapies have largely replaced the use of estrogens in recurrent breast cancer.

- Palliation is the principal goal of endocrine therapy in recurrent breast cancer.

Indications for Endocrine Therapy (Jones & Buzdar, 2004)

- Selection of patients for endocrine therapy is individualized.
- Patients most likely to respond to endocrine therapy include the following:
  1. Those with ER-positive and/or PR-positive tumor
  2. Disease-free interval greater than 2 years
  3. Metastatic disease confined to bone and soft tissue only
  4. Asymptomatic visceral disease
  5. Good response to past endocrine therapy
  6. Postmenopausal or late premenopausal status
  7. Prior response to endocrine therapy
- NCCN guidelines for endocrine treatment of systemic disease can be accessed online at www.nccn.org/professionals/physician_gls/PDF/breast.pdf.
- Endocrine therapy differs between postmenopausal and premenopausal women.

Table 14-1 lists the possible endocrine therapies based on menopausal status recommended by NCCN guidelines.

Table 14-2 lists the class of endocrine therapy used in recurrent breast cancer.

See Chapter 11 for a discussion of hormonal therapy for primary breast cancer. These agents include tamoxifen, anastrozole, letrozole, and exemestane.

TABLE 14-1

Endocrine Therapies Related to Menopausal Status

Menopausal Status	Endocrine Therapy
Postmenopausal	
Prior endocrine therapy within past 12 months	Nonsteroidal aromatase inhibitor (i.e., anastrozole or letrozole)
Endocrine therapy naïve or are more than 12 months from previous endocrine therapy	Either tamoxifen or nonsteroidal aromatase inhibitor
Premenopausal	
Prior endocrine therapy within past 12 months	Surgical or radiotherapeutic oophorectomy or leuteinizing hormone-releasing hormone (LHRH) agonist with or without an antiestrogen
Endocrine therapy naive	Antiestrogen with or without LHRH agonist

TABLE 14-2

Endocrine Therapy in Recurrent Breast Cancer

Category of Endocrine Therapy	Agent
Selective Estrogen Receptor Modulator (SERM)	Tamoxifen
	Toremifene
Steroidal antiestrogen	Fulvestrant
Nonsteroidal aromatase inhibitors	Anastrozole
	Letrozole
Steroidal aromatase inhibitor	Exemestane
Luteinizing hormone-releasing hormone (LHRH) agonist	Leuprolide/ goserelin
Progestin	Megestrol acetate

Types of Endocrine Therapy

The following is a discussion of the agents tamoxifen, toremifene, fulvestrant, aromatese inhibitors, progestins, and LHRH agonists used in recurrent breast cancer.

Tamoxifen

- Synthetic nonsteroidal triphenylethylene antiestrogen that binds to ER.

- Demonstrates mixed agonist/antagonist activity.

- Patients achieve good palliation.

- Mean time to disease progression for patients on tamoxifen is 6 months, with a duration of response of 12 to 18 months and up to several years.

- Serious complications include thromboembolic events, endometrial cancer, pulmonary embolism, and cataracts. Side effects include hot flashes, nausea, and vaginal discharge, as well as potential depression.

Toremifene (Pagani, et al., 2004)

1. Is a SERM that is used as an alternative to tamoxifen
2. Has a side effect profile similar to tamoxifen including hot flashes, vaginal discharge, bleeding, irregular menses, nausea and increased risk of endometrial cancer and thromboembolic events
3. Has cross resistance with tamoxifen

Fulvestrant (Buzdar, 2004; Dienger, 2004; Howell, et al., 2004; Johnston, 2004)

1. Is a pure steroidal antiestrogen that binds to the ER of the nuclear cell membrane. It blocks estrogen-regulated gene transcription and causes a loss of the ER protein from the cell (also known as ER down regulation).
2. Has no estrogenic effect and thus there is no increased risk of endometrial cancer with its use
3. Does not cross the blood brain barrier, leading to a decrease in the incidence of hot flashes

4. Is contraindicated in patients with bleeding problems, thrombocytopenia, or patients on anticoagulants

5. Cannot be absorbed orally. It is administered as a monthly intramuscular injection of 250 mg

6. May be used for patients who may be noncompliant with daily medication

Aromatase Inhibitors (Grana, 2004; Sokolowicz & Gradishar, 2004; Choueiri, et al., 2004)

- In postmenopausal women, estrogen synthesis in nongonadal sites increases. Peripheral tissue depends on the aromatization of androgenic precursors of adrenal origin (testosterone and androstenedione) to generate estradiol and estrone.

- Aromatase is responsible for converting androgens to estrogens.

- Aromatase inhibitors suppress postmenopausal estrogen by inhibiting the aromatase enzyme.

- Side effects include fatigue, headache, hot flashes, and gastrointestinal disturbance (e.g., nausea, vomiting, diarrhea).

- There are two classes of aromatase inhibitors:
    1. Nonsteroidal aromatase inhibitors are anastrozole and letrozole.
    2. The steroidal aromatase inhibitor is exemestane. Exemestane has no cross-resistance with nonsteroidal aromatase inhibitors.

Luteinizing Hormone-Releasing Hormone Agonists (Aebi & Castiglione-Gertsch, 2003; Sainsbury, 2003)

- LHRH agonists are an alternative to oophorectomy for premenopausal women.

- Goserelin and leuprolide are peptide analogues of LHRH that are up to 100 times more potent than the natural hormone.

- LHRH agonists stimulate follicle-stimulating hormone and luteinizing hormone secretion and affect the pituitary ovarian axis, with a resulting fall in estrogen to menopausal levels.

- LHRH agonists have been combined with tamoxifen as first-line therapy in premenopausal women with metastatic disease, but the overall survival benefit is small.

Progestins

- Endocrine therapy with progestins such as megestrol acetate are used when further endocrine therapy is needed after disease progression.

- Mechanism of action is unknown but may involve direct action on the cell mediated through progesterone and androgen receptor sites.

- Side effects include hypertension, weight gain, fluid retention, vaginal bleeding, and thromboembolic events.

Management of Side Effects (Dienger, 2004)

- Nurses often regard endocrine therapy as somewhat "benign," compared with chemotherapy. However, patients experience side effects and are facing metastatic disease.

- Side effect profiles vary across the different endocrine therapies.

- Tamoxifen is associated with agonist and antagonist activity and include hot flashes, amenorrhea, vaginal bleeding, weight gain, fluid retention, nausea and vomiting, flare reaction, increased risk of endometrial cancer, and thrombosis.

- The aromatase inhibitors and fulvestrant have a similar side effect profile to one another and include headache, joint pain, hot flashes, and nausea and vomiting.

- Hot flashes are a major source of distress. The reader is referred to Chapter 19 for further discussion of the management of hot flashes.

REFERENCES

Aebi, S., & Castiglione-Gertsch, M. (2003). Adjuvant endocrine therapy for the very young patients. *Breast, 12*(6), 509–515.

Buzdar, A. U. (2004). Fulvestrant: A new type of estrogen receptor antagonist for the treatment of advanced breast cancer. *Drugs Today (Barc), 40*(9), 751–764.

Choueiri, T. K., Alemany, C. A., Abou-Jawde, R. M., & Budd, G. T. (2004). Role of aromatase inhibitors in the treatment of breast cancer. *Clinical Therapeutics, 26*(8), 1199–1214.

Dienger, J. (2004). Hormonal therapy in advanced and metastatic disease. In K. H. Dow (Ed.), *Contemporary issues in breast cancer: A nursing persective* (2nd ed., pp. 175–187). Sudbury, MA: Jones & Bartlett.

Ellis, M., Hayes, D., & Lippman, M. (2004). Treatment of metastatic breast cancer. In J. R. Harris, M. Lippman, M. Morrow, & C. K. Osborne (Eds.), *Diseases of the breast* (3rd ed., pp. 1101–1159). Philadelphia: Lippincott Williams & Wilkins.

Grana, G. (2004). Shifting paradigms in hormonal therapy for breast cancer. *Cancer Biology and Therapy, 3*(9), 797–805.

Howell, A., Robertson, J. F., Abram, P., Lichinitser, M. R., Elledge, R., Bajetta, E., et al. (2004). Comparison of fulvestrant versus tamoxifen for the treatment of advanced breast cancer in postmenopausal women previously untreated with endocrine therapy: A multinational, double-blind, randomized trial. *Journal of Clinical Oncology, 22*(9), 1605–1613.

Johnston, S. (2004). Fulvestrant and the sequential endocrine cascade for advanced breast cancer. *British Journal of Cancer, 90 Suppl 1*, S15–18.

Jones, K. L., & Buzdar, A. U. (2004). A review of adjuvant hormonal therapy in breast cancer. *Endocrine-Related Cancer, 11*(3), 391–406.

Pagani, O., Gelber, S., Price, K., Zahrieh, D., Gelber, R., Simoncini, E., et al. (2004). Toremifene and tamoxifen are equally effective for early-stage breast cancer: First results of International Breast Cancer Study Group Trials 12-93 and 14-93. *Annals of Oncology, 15*(12), 1749–1759.

Sainsbury, R. (2003). Ovarian ablation as a treatment for breast cancer. *Surgical Oncology, 12*(4), 241–250.

Sokolowicz, L. E., & Gradishar, W. J. (2004). Implications of first-line adjuvant treatment with aromatase inhibitors in recurrent metastatic breast cancer. *Clinical Breast Cancer, 5 Suppl 1*, S24–30.

PART IV

*Quality-of-Life Issues
in Breast Cancer*

CHAPTER FIFTEEN

Cancer-Related Fatigue and Sleep Disturbance

Cancer-Related Fatigue (Broekel, et al., 1998; Berger & Higginbotham, 2000; Velez-Barone, 2004)

- According to the NCCN Practice Guidelines, the definition of cancer-related fatigue (CRF) is "a persistent, subjective sense of tiredness related to cancer or cancer treatment that interferes with usual functioning."

- CRF is the most common side effect of treatment requiring a multidisciplinary approach to assessment and management.

- CRF is not a life-threatening condition, but needs prompt treatment because CRF can

  1. Influence one's sense of well-being and quality of life

2.   Change the activities of daily living

3.   Affect relationships with family and friends

4.   Change one's work-related activities

5.   Affect compliance with treatment

- NCCN guidelines for the assessment and management of CRF can be accessed online at www.nccn.org/professionals/physician_gls/PDF/fatigue.pdf.

- Screening for fatigue should occur on a regular basis using a severity score of 0–10 with 0 representing no fatigue and 10 representing the worst fatigue one can imagine.

- Severity of CRF is categorized as mild (1–3), moderate (4–6), and severe (7–10). Recommendations for treatment are based on these categories.

- Multiple factors contribute to CRF and include

  Pain

  Emotional distress

  Sleep disturbance

  Anemia

  Nutritional imbalance

  Activity level

  Comorbidities such as infection, cardiac, pulmonary, renal, hepatic, neurologic, and endocrine dysfunction

- NCCN distinguishes the treatable contributing factors as pain, emotional distress, anemia, sleep disturbance, nutritional imbalance, activity level, and comorbidities.

- Etiology of fatigue in breast cancer are also multifactorial.

- Surgical intervention:

  Postoperative fatigue may be self-limiting.

  Other side effects from surgery, such as limited range of arm motion and pain, may increase the experience of fatigue.

  Acute and chronic lymphedema may contribute to fatigue.

- Radiation therapy:

  Pattern of fatigue in radiation therapy is progressive and increases during the course of treatment.

  Radiation side effects, such as skin reactions, may contribute to fatigue patterns, even when there is no change in red blood cell count.

- Adjuvant chemotherapy (Broekel, et al., 1998; Berger & Higginbotham, 2000):

  Treatment-related side effects, such as neutropenia, nausea, vomiting, weight gain, skin changes, nutritional pattern changes, and stomatitis, contribute to fatigue.

  Symptom cluster of sleep disturbances, anxiety, and depression may also contribute to the experience of fatigue.

Interventions for CRF

- Patient and family education and counseling regarding known patterns of fatigue include daily self-monitoring of fatigue levels.

- Practice energy conservation.
    1. Set priorities and pace activities, distinguish between required and nonessential activities, periods of rest, and relaxation.
    2. Determine level of attentional fatigue and plan attention-restoring activities.
    3. Plan and pace activities.
- Promote rest and sleep.
- Nutritional evaluation:

    Weight gain and weight loss

    Caloric intake

    Fluid and electrolyte balance
- Behavioral interventions (Servaes, et al., 2002):

    May be directed at balanced activity levels, restorative therapy, sleep hygiene, stress management, relaxation activities, and social support.

    Relaxation techniques, biofeedback, and massage therapy have been suggested and may be a promising intervention, but there are no controlled studies available to evaluate their effectiveness.
- Pharmacologic interventions:

    Recombinant human erythropoietin (epoetin alfa) is a recognized and effective approach to treating anemia that may contribute to CRF.

    Psychostimulants such as methylphenidate has been used for CRF.

Antidepressant therapy also used. Important to distinguish differences between CRF and depression.

- Table 15-1 outlines the differences between fatigue and depression.

Exercise as an Intervention for Fatigue

- NCCN guidelines recommend exercise as the non-pharmacologic intervention having the strongest evidence of effectiveness with CRF.

- Types of exercise include home-based walking programs and structured exercise programs in the community.

- A self-paced walking program allows for periods of decreased performance due to effects of the disease or treatment. Self-paced walking exercise program should be modest enough for the individual to feel successful.

- A review of studies indicate significantly lower levels of fatigue in individuals who exercise, compared

TABLE 15-1

Differences Between Fatigue and Depression

Fatigue	Depression
Identifiable cause, such as anemia and infection	No identified cause
Cause may be treatable	No discernible pattern of fatigue
Pattern is related to cancer treatment	Intensity, pattern, and duration of sadness meet standard definition of depression

with randomized control subjects. Study outcomes also demonstrate increased performance, decreased anxiety and depression, and improved quality of life.

Sample Exercise Program

- General program

  1. Begin range of motion (ROM)/flexibility exercises and muscle strengthening, to maximize joint ROM and muscle endurance.

  2. Follow by submaximal aerobic exercise to enhance cardiopulmonary endurance.

- The three basic components of an exercise program are frequency, intensity, and duration.

  Frequency involves the number of exercises performed or the number of walks per week.

  1. *Beginning walking exercise may be three to four times a week.*

  2. *More frequent, short-time periods are recommended rather than less frequent but longer periods of exercise.*

  Intensity refers to how difficult the exercise is; difficulty being determined by the heart rate.

  1. Women in an exercise program should be taught to take their pulse for 60 seconds while resting, to assess rate and rhythm.

  2. During exercise, the peak pulse just before the cool-down period is best measured by counting the pulse for 6 seconds and multiplying by 10.

3. Because the pulse drops quickly when the individual stops exercising to measure it, the 6-second monitoring check best captures the peak pulse rate.

4. As an intensity guide, the rating of perceived exertion is a helpful adjunct to heart rate.

Duration: The length of the exercise period is initially determined by the usual activity level of the individual.

1. Begin gradually with a 5- or 10-minute brisk walk, always beginning (to warm up) and ending (to cool down) with several minutes of slow walking.

Precautions and Contraindications in an Exercise Program

- Precautions
    1. Wear comfortable, supportive shoes made specifically for walking or running.
    2. Exercise in safe areas and preferably with an exercise partner.
    3. Carry an emergency card and identification while running.
    4. Keep hydrated.
- Contraindications to Exercise
    1. No exercise is recommended on the days of chemotherapy administration.

2. No exercise is recommended before blood drawing to check laboratory values.

3. No exercise is recommended if any of the following laboratory values are present:

   - White blood cell count less than 3,000 µL
   - Absolute neutrophil count less than 2,500 µL
   - Hemoglobin/hematocrit less than 10 g/dL
   - Platelet count less than 25,000 µL

4. Do not recommend exercise if there is metastatic bone involvement of greater than 25% of the cortex.

5. High-impact aerobics are contraindicated during chemotherapy and in recurrent disease and in the presence of a fever.

6. Recommend resumption of exercise carefully following illness, surgery, or new treatment protocols.

Adherence to an Exercise Program

- Exercise is a learned behavior; the first goal should be to establish the habit of exercise.

- Incorporate effective behavioral strategies to encourage adherence.

- Women with breast cancer are often highly motivated to do whatever they can to improve their health.

- Regular reinforcement by supportive friends and family members and members of the health care team can help sustain the patient's commitment.

- Encourage the patient to keep an exercise diary, which offers a patient the reward of seeing her progress over time and may help reinforce the exercise habit.

- Encourage the patient to exercise with a committed friend or family member.

- Some individuals prefer group exercise and find that this enhances their adherence.

- Exercise should be enjoyable; examples include walking, jogging, swimming, and biking.

- Schedule the exercise period as a part of one's daily activities and at a convenient time and location.

Sleep Disturbance (Berger & Farr, 1999; Berger, et al., 2003; Fortner, et al., 2002; Koopman, et al., 2002)

- Sleep disturbance and mood changes often accompany fatigue.

- Sleep problems are a common side effect gaining increased clinical and research attention for interventions.

- Risk factors for sleep problems in women with metastatic breast cancer include depression, pain, bony metastasis, and lack of social support.

- Sleep problems are categorized as insomnia (inability to sleep) or hypersomnia (inability to maintain wakefulness).

- Chronic sleep problems may lead to difficulty concentrating or paying attention, irritability, and depression.

- Assessment of sleep disturbance is complex.

  Determine the differences in the current level of sleep patterns, compared with that before treatment.

  Evaluate the quality and quantity of sleep since the cancer diagnosis.

  What are the patterns of insomnia (sleep onset, awakenings)?

  What are the present presleep routines? Daily activities?

  What are the environmental considerations in sleep (noise, light, room temperature)?

  Are there any physiologic problems present that can interfere with sleep such as pain, dyspnea, hot flashes?

  What food and medications may be interfering with sleep? These might include caffeine or alcohol.

  What are the emotional factors that may affect sleep?

- Management of sleep disturbance

  Keep a sleep log to record the time of sleep onset, duration of sleep, sleep habits, frequency and reason for awakening, naps, and use of sleep aids.

- There are two categories of management: nonpharmacologic and pharmacologic.

  1. Nonpharmacologic management

     Establish a sleep ritual: A time for sleep and awakening every day.

     Avoid stimulants (e.g., caffeine, chocolate, nicotine), alcohol, heavy meals, and exercise just prior to sleep.

Take a warm bath or shower before sleep.

Exercise regularly to improve sleep.

Control of other symptoms and side effects of treatment can be done using: behavioral relaxation, including progressive muscle relaxation training, passive muscle relaxation training, meditation, hypnosis, and guided imagery, cognitive control techniques, including counting, cognitive refocusing, guided imagery, and ocular relaxation

2. Pharmacologic intervention

   Benzodiazepines

   Nonbenzodiazepine (chloral hydrate)

   Nonbarbiturates

   Antidepressants

REFERENCES

Berger, A. M., & Farr, L. (1999). The influence of daytime inactivity and nighttime restlessness on cancer-related fatigue. *Oncology Nursing Forum, 26*(10), 1663–1671.

Berger, A. M., & Higginbotham, P. (2000). Correlates of fatigue during and following adjuvant breast cancer chemotherapy: A pilot study. *Oncology Nursing Forum, 27*(9), 1443–1448.

Berger, A. M., VonEssen, S., Kuhn, B. R., Piper, B. F., Agrawal, S., Lynch, J. C., et al. (2003). Adherence, sleep, and fatigue outcomes after adjuvant breast cancer chemotherapy: Results of a feasibility intervention study. *Oncology Nursing Forum, 30*(3), 513–522.

Broekel, J. A., Jacobsen, P. B., Horton, J., et al. (1998). Characteristics and correlates of fatigue after adjuvant chemotherapy for breast cancer. *Journal of Clinical Oncology, 16*, 1689–1696.

Fortner, B. V., Stepanski, E. J., Wang, S. C., Kasprowicz, S., & Durrence, H. H. (2002). Sleep and quality of life in breast cancer patients. *Journal of Pain Symptom Management, 24*(5), 471–480.

Koopman, C., Nouriani, B., Erickson, V., Anupindi, R., Butler, L. D., Bachmann, M. H., et al. (2002). Sleep disturbances in women with metastatic breast cancer. *The Breast Journal, 8*(6), 362–370.

Mock, V., Atkinson, A., Barsevick, A., Cella, D., Cimprich, B., Cleeland, C., et al. (2000). NCCN practice guidelines for cancer-related fatigue. *Oncology (Huntington), 14*(11A), 151–161.

Servaes, P., Prins, J., Verhagen, S., & Bleijenberg, G. (2002). Fatigue after breast cancer and in chronic fatigue syndrome: similarities and differences. *Journal of Psychosomatic Research, 52*(6), 453–459.

Velez-Barone, G. (2004). Fatigue, sleep disturbance and pain. In K. H. Dow (Ed.), *Contemporary issues in breast cancer: A nursing persective* (2nd ed., pp. 198–207). Sudbury, MA: Jones & Bartlett.

CHAPTER SIXTEEN

Lymphedema

Overview and Definition

- Lymphedema is an abnormal collection of excessive tissue proteins, edema, chronic inflammation, and fibrosis that occurs from an imbalance between fluid deposited in tissue and the ability of the lymphatic system to handle the fluid. It is the result of a functional overload of the lymphatic system in which lymph volume exceeds transport capabilities.

Problems with Lymphedema

- Breast cancer is the leading cause of lymphedema (Armer, 2004; Hull, 2000).

- Lymphedema is a recognized complication of breast cancer treatment that affects approximately 20% of patients (Petrek, et al., 2000).

- With lymphedema, there is a significant and persistent swelling in the affected arm. The swelling is related to accumulation of protein-rich fluid.

- Restriction of arm movement can limit activities of daily living, affect functional abilities, and interfere with the quality of life.

- There is no cure for lymphedema. Thus, efforts are aimed at prevention, early recognition, and prompt treatment.

- Unmanaged lymphedema is associated with additional health problems including cellulitis, lymphadenitis, open wounds, infection, and septicemia.

- Lymphedema is often underrecognized and undertreated for several reasons including:

   1. Lymphedema has not been considered a life-threatening side effect.

   2. Lymphedema onset is insidious, occurring over several years.

Pathophysiology of Lymphedema in Breast Cancer

- Lymphedema associated with breast cancer is considered secondary lymphedema caused by mechanical obstruction of lymphatic channels after surgery and/or radiation therapy (Goffman, et al., 2004). See Chapter 6 on surgical techniques for additional information about axillary lymph node dissection (ALND).

   ALND of level I, II, and III nodes contributes significantly to the development of lymphedema.

1. Level I nodes are located at the tail of the breast.

2. Level II nodes are closest to the breast and drain the breast area.

3. Level III nodes are located between the pectoralis muscle along subscapular vessels and the chest wall.

Sentinel lymph node biopsy (SLNB) is increasingly used as an alternative to ALND. SLNB is associated with a decreased risk and incidence of lymphedema, but does not eliminate the risk altogether (Armer, et al., 2004).

- Radiation therapy to the axilla increases the risk of lymphedema.

Incidence of lymphedema is greatest when both ALND and axillary radiation are performed.

Although lymphatic vessels are resistant to radiation, lymph nodes are sensitive and go through a process of reduced lymphocytes, fatty tissue replacement, and localized fibrosis.

- Additional risk factors for lymphedema may include (Erickson, et al., 2001; National Cancer Institute, 2004):

Postoperative infection.

Advanced cancer-causing bulky lymphadenopathy.

Obesity and poor nutritional status that may increase the risk of delayed wound healing.

Individual differences in lymphatic anatomy and physiology.

Classification of Lymphedema

- Lymphedema is classified as either primary or secondary.

  1. Primary lymphedema is caused by abnormalities in the lymphatic fluid or is a congenital and rare condition.

  2. Secondary lymphedema is caused by an obstruction or interruption of the lymphatic system as a result of cancer, trauma, infection, and/or scarring. Lymphedema associated with breast cancer is considered secondary lymphedema.

- Lymphedema may either be acute or chronic.

  1. *Acute* lymphedema lasts between 3 and 6 months and has a pitting quality.

     Excess fluid is accommodated by a large subcutaneous tissue space that can expand.

     Noticeable fluctuations in arm size are typical with the largest increase noted at night.

     - There are four different forms of acute lymphedema (Armer, 2004):

       1. Transient and mild lymphedema occurs within a few days of surgery with the affected area feeling warm and red. Transient lymphedema is not generally painful. This form of lymphedema responds to limb elevation and gentle muscle pumping.

2. Acute lymphangitis or phlebitis may occur within 6 to 8 weeks after surgery. The affected area feels warm, tender, and red. This form of lymphedema responds to elevation and anti-inflammatory medication.

3. Erysipeloid lymphedema occurs after an insect bite, minor injury, or burn. The affected area feels warm to hot and is very tender. This form of lymphedema responds to limb elevation and antibiotics. No compression pumping or wrapping is recommended.

4. The fourth type of lymphedema occurs insidiously about 18 to 24 months after treatment. The affected area is generally **not** red, but there is aching and skin discomfort associated with this condition.

2. *Chronic* lymphedema lasts longer than 6 months.

   Chronic lymphedema is the most difficult to manage due to the related pathophysiology where a deficient lymphatic system of the limb cannot compensate for the increased demand for fluid drainage.

   The affected skin becomes hard, thick, and brawny in appearance.

   Change occurs over time, as fluid becomes embedded in subcutaneous connective tissues, restricting joint movement, and gradually causing edema to be nonpitting.

Severity of Lymphedema

- Lymphedema is further categorized according to severity: mild (Grade 1); moderate (Grade II); or severe (Grade III).

  1. *Grade I:* Pitting occurs by applying pressure. Edema reverses with limb elevation.

  2. *Grade II:* Edema becomes larger and harder and does not pit under pressure.

  3. *Grade III:* Swelling worsens and skin changes occur; skin becomes thick and develops folds, with elephantiasis.

NCI Classification of Secondary Lymphedema

- The NCI developed a clinical classification and management guideline for the treatment of secondary lymphedema in an effort to address and standardize previous lack of criteria.

- There continues to be a lack of uniform diagnostic criteria for lymphedema. Objective criteria are based on circumferential or volumetric measurement.

- The information can be accessed online at www.cancer.gov/cancertopics/pdq/supportive care/lymphedema/healthprofessional/.

  1+: *Edema that is barely detectable.*

  2+: *A slight indentation is visible when the skin is depressed.*

  3+: *A deeper fingerprint returns to normal in 5 to 30 seconds.*

  4+: *The extremity may be 1.5 to 2 times normal size.*

Symptoms that May Occur with Lymphedema

- About 50% of patients report a feeling of heaviness or fullness in the extremity.

- Pain

  Pain is related to nerve damage during surgery; postmastectomy pain syndrome.

  Stretching of tissue accommodates the build-up of lymph fluid.

  When the fluid increases, the arm becomes visibly swollen and feels heavy, with an increase in arm size.

- Restriction in range of motion (ROM) in the ipsilateral arm

  ROM is the result of tissue manipulation and positioning during surgery.

  Lymphedema also causes ROM restrictions in the shoulder, elbow, and wrist.

- Sensation changes

  Sensation changes may be related to surgical incision or to nerve irritation or injury during ALND.

  Sensations include phantom breast sensations, numbness, hyperesthesias, and "pins-and-needles" sensations.

  Dysesthesia is described as a cutting or burning pain.

Diagnosis of Lymphedema

- Women often present with a feeling of heaviness, fullness, or tightness in clothing or jewelry.

- Physical examination with findings of a greater than 2-cm difference between affected and contralateral limb circumferences have been used. However, anatomical variations and handedness may make these differences clinically meaningless.

- The NCI suggests that other measures include water displacement measurement 15 cm above the epicondyle may be a good objective criterion.

- Indirect volume measurements may also provide suitable follow-up measurement (Meijer, et al., 2004).

- Optimally, sequential measurement over time with a baseline pretreatment measure may provide good objective information.

- Lack of agreement about standard measurement with acceptable reliability and validity, lack of uniform definition, and evaluation of treatments contribute to problems in the diagnosis of lymphedema.

Prevention of Lymphedema

- Prevention is the major goal, because there is no cure for lymphedema.

- Focus of prevention is minimizing injury or damage to the involved extremity.

- The NCI recommends the following considerations for prevention and control of lymphedema:

  1. Keep the arm elevated above the level of the heart whenever possible.

2. Clean and lubricate the skin daily.

3. Avoid injury of the affected arm. Use an electric razor for shaving, wear gardening and cooking gloves, maintain good nail care, and do not cut the cuticles.

4. Avoid constrictive pressure on the arm. Wear loose jewelry and clothing with no constricting bands, carry the handbag on the opposite arm, and do not use blood pressure cuffs on the vulnerable limb.

5. Monitor the arm for signs of infection.

6. Practice the prescribed exercises as instructed.

7. Keep regular follow-up appointments.

8. Observe the limbs daily for sign of problems.

- In addition, the 18-step recommendations for prevention of lymphedema to the upper extremity recommended by National Lymphedema Network can be accessed online at www.lymphnet.org/prevention.html (Thiadens, 1999).

Management of Lymphedema

- Management of lymphedema consists of three major strategies: mechanical, pharmacologic, and nutritional.

  1. Mechanical interventions include elevation of the affected limb; manual lymphatic drainage, compression bandages, and custom fitted pressure-graded garments (McNeely, et al., 2004).

Cochrane database review found that compression bandages were effective and that manual lymph drainage (MLD) provides no extra benefit. However, meta-analysis of current data could not be performed because of poor quality of studies (Badger, et al., 2004).

Several strategies have been combined into a program called complex physical therapy (CPT) or complex decongestive therapy consisting of manual lymphedema treatment, compression wrapping, individualized exercises, skin care, and an additional maintenance program.

CPT is an effective approach to managing lymphedema that is not responsive to standard compression therapy.

CPT is done by trained lymphedema therapists.

- Four components include:
    1. Skin care
    2. Massage
    3. Compression bandaging
    4. Exercise

Two phases of CPT include the first phase lasting 4 to 6 weeks to establish lymphedema reduction and the second phase involving maintenance.

2. Pharmacologic Management

Antibiotics are used to treat and prevent cellulitis and lymphangitis.

Pain management with nonopioid analgesics and transcutaneous nerve stimulation (TENS) may be used.

Other drug interventions that have not shown benefit include diuretics and anticoagulants.

3. Nutritional Management

Patients should be encouraged to eat protein-rich foods and supplements.

Hypoalbuminemia allows fluid to pass into interstitial tissues with excess protein. Thus, serum albumin levels need to be maintained above 2.5 g/dL.

Psychosocial Issues

- Lymphedema can be disfiguring, painful, and interferes with daily functioning. Thus, breast cancer survivors may experience depression and anxiety.

- Body-image concerns relate to the appearance of the arm and its function.

- Treatments for management of lymphedema are time consuming and may increase breast cancer survivors' feelings of social isolation.

- Diminished quality of life is associated with lymphedema.

Nursing Management of Lymphedema
(Armer, 2004)

- Armer (2004) identifies several excellent strategies for nursing management of lymphedema. The strategies are reproduced here and include:

1. Initiate education on lymphedema prevention at the preoperative visit and review the patient's understanding at regular follow-up visits.

2. Ensure that the patient has written guidelines and educational materials for future reference.

3. Review lymphedema pathophysiology and steps to prevention.

4. Instruct the patient on establishing routine circumferential measurements of both the affected and the nonaffected limb at easy-to-find personal landmarks.

5. Ask patients about lymphedema or limb swelling or other signs and symptoms; patients may not volunteer information unless asked directly.

6. Monitor patients closely when lymphedema occurs; evaluate and manage the symptoms.

7. Facilitate a referral to a certified manual lymph drainage therapist for assessment, intensive treatment, and instruction on self-management.

8. Instruct the patient to report any rash, redness, tenderness, swelling of the affected area (hand, arm, breast and/or scapular region), and increased temperature immediately.

9. Be alert to the risk of repeated infections in the patient who has experienced a single infection.

10. Do not dismiss even a seemingly minor injury.

11. Encourage a well-balanced, protein-sufficient diet; review nutritional status and lab work routinely for lypoalbuminemia.

12. Assess psychosocial concerns as well as physical and functional changes.

13. Explore perceived barriers to self-management and compliance and provide resources for problem solving.

14. Assess patients in assessing personal short-term and long-term goals and placing self-management actions in the context of these self-concordant goals.

15. Suggest that patients wear a medical alert bracelet.

REFERENCES

Armer, J. (2004). Lymphedema. In K.H. Dow (Ed.), *Contemporary issues in breast cancer: A nursing persective* (2nd ed., pp. 209–229). Sudbury, MA: Jones & Bartlett.

Armer, J., Fu, M. R., Wainstock, J. M., Zagar, E., & Jacobs, L. K. (2004). Lymphedema following breast cancer treatment, including sentinel lymph node biopsy. *Lymphology, 37*(2), 73–91.

Badger, C., Preston, N., Seers, K., & Mortimer, P. (2004). Physical therapies for reducing and controlling lymphoedema of the limbs. *Cochrane Database of Systematic Reviews, (4),* CD003141.

Erickson, V. S., Pearson, M. L., Ganz, P. A., Adams, J., & Kahn, K. L. (2001). Arm edema in breast cancer patients. *Journal of the National Cancer Institute, 93*(2), 96–111.

Goffman, T. E., Laronga, C., Wilson, L., & Elkins, D. (2004). Lymphedema of the arm and breast in irradiated breast cancer patients: Risks in an era of dramatically changing axillary surgery. *The Breast Journal, 10*(5), 405–411.

Hull, M. M. (2000). Lymphedema in women treated for breast cancer. *Seminars in Oncology Nursing, 16*(3), 226–237.

McNeely, M. L., Magee, D. J., Lees, A. W., Bagnall, K. M., Haykowsky, M., & Hanson, J. (2004). The addition of manual lymph drainage to compression therapy for breast cancer related lymphedema: A randomized controlled trial. *Breast Cancer Research and Treatment, 86*(2), 95–106.

Meijer, R. S., Rietman, J. S., Geertzen, J. H., Bosmans, J. C., & Dijkstra, P. U. (2004). Validity and intra- and interobserver reliability of an indirect volume measurements in patients with upper extremity lymphedema. *Lymphology, 37*(3), 127–133.

National Cancer Institute. (2004). *Lymphedema (PDQ) Health Professional Version*. Retrieved November 27, 2004, from www.cancer.gov/cancertopics/pdq/supportivecare/ lymphedema/healthprofessional

Petrek, J. A., Pressman, P. I., & Smith, R. A. (2000). Lymphedema: Current issues in research and management. *CA: A Cancer Journal for Clinicians, 50*, 292.

Thiadens, S. (1999). *18 steps to prevention for arm lymphedema*. Retrieved November 27, 2004, from www.lymphnet.org/ prevention.html

CHAPTER SEVENTEEN

Menopausal Symptoms

Introduction

- Menopausal symptoms occurring as a result of breast cancer treatment have a significant effect on the quality of life of women (Swain, et al., 1999; Carpenter & Elam, 2004).

- Assessment and management of menopausal symptoms are important because of the increasing number of breast cancer survivors who are living longer with chronic disease and the aging population.

Menopause

- The definition of *menopause* is the cessation of menses or amenorrhea occurring after 12 months or more that is not associated with pathologic or physiologic cause (Utian, 2001).

- The definition of *induced menopause* is the absence of menses after either surgical removal of both ovaries or iatrogenic ablation of ovarian function that may be caused by chemotherapy or radiation therapy (Utian, 2001).

- Perimenopausal is the period of time immediately prior to menopause.

- Premenopausal is the entire reproductive period before perimenopause.

- The average age of occurrence of natural menopause is 51 to 52 years (range: 40–60 years).

- Premature menopause is defined as occurring prior to the age of 40 years.

Changes Occurring During Menopause

- The transition from regular menstrual cycles to amenorrhea include several morphologic change in the ovaries as a result of changes in hormonal levels.

- Ovaries become smaller, fibrotic, and devoid of any functional follicle.

- Estradiol, the dominant source of estrogen for the premenopausal woman, dramatically declines.

- Estrone becomes the principal source of estrogen for the postmenopausal woman. Estrone is derived from the peripheral conversion of androstenedione.

- Levels of gonadotrophins (FSH and LH) rise significantly after menopause due to estrogen loss.

- The decline in circulating estrogen affects several target tissues in the body.

Menopause and Cancer

- Women with breast cancer are at increased risk of developing menopausal symptoms.

- Breast cancer survivors are not likely to receive hormone replacement therapy (HRT) for managing hot flashes. HRT is contraindicated in women with a history of breast cancer. In addition, only a small percentage of breast cancer survivors are willing to take HRT.

- Breast cancer survivors may have artificially induced menopause as a result of chemotherapy, radiation therapy, surgery, and/or tamoxifen therapy.

  Radiation therapy to the ovaries will induce amenorrhea.

  Surgical removal of the ovaries (i.e., oophorectomy) will lead to menopausal symptoms.

  Chemotherapy produces gonadal toxicity (i.e., cyclophosphamide).

  Endocrine therapy with tamoxifen and the aromatase inhibitors increases the risk of hot flashes.

- There is an increased problem of hot flashes in women with breast cancer (Carpenter, 2000).

  Women may have been on HRT previously but must discontinue it after a breast cancer diagnosis and thus precipitate or exacerbate hot flashes (Snyder, et al., 1998).

  Hot flashes and other menopausal symptoms are more frequent, severe, bothersome, and disruptive in women with breast cancer, compared with naturally

> *premenopausal, perimenopausal, and post-menopausal women (Carpenter, 2001).*
>
> *Hot flashes also can occur with tamoxifen therapy.*
>
> *Disruption of circadian rhythms of hormone and body temperature may also affect the severity of hot flashes.*

Targets Affected by Menopause

- Vasomotor
- Skeletal system
- Cardiovascular system
- Urogenital tract

Vasomotor Symptoms: Hot Flashes

- Hot flashes are the most frequently occurring symptom of menopause, with up to 85% of women experiencing hot flashes.

- Etiology of hot flashes is unknown but consists of both a subjective and physiologic component with estrogen withdrawal and disruption of thermoregulation and neuroendocrine pathways.

- Hot flashes are also thought to result from increases in core body temperature that occur within a reduced thermoregulatory null zone (Freedman, 1998; Freedman & Krell, 1999). The thermoregulatory null zone is defined as the threshold between sweating (high end) and shivering (low end). If the thermoregulatory null zone is decreased (Figure 17-1), an increase in core body temperature can lead to a ceiling effect of sweating, and a decrease in core body temperature can lead to a floor effect of shivering (Figure 17-2).

- Symptoms are unique to the individual.

  Vary from transient episodes of feelings of warmth to episodes of intense overheating

  May be accompanied by sweats, palpitations, anxiety, and chills

  May report experiencing a premonition or aura right before the hot flash

  Heart rate and skin blood flow increase, and distribution of the heat sensation is to the upper body

  Hot flashes occur at various times during a 24-hour period, with no particular established pattern

Figure 17-1 and 17-2
Fluctuations in Core Body Temperature and the Thermoregulatory Null Zone

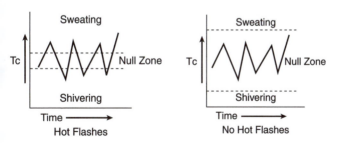

Tc = core body temperature
Source: Figures reproduced from Carpenter, J. and Elam, J. (2004). Menopausal symptoms. *Contemporary Issues in Breast Cancer, 235*(12).

- Key factor is the withdrawal of estrogen, not low estrogen level.
- Other precipitating factors that increase the likelihood of hot flashes include ambient temperature, hot drinks and food, alcohol, caffeine, and emotional distress.

Pharmacologic Management of Hot Flashes (Cobleigh, 2000)

- Venlafaxine is an antidepressant that affects serotonin and norepinephrine reuptake and has been effective in reducing hot flashes in a placebo-controlled clinical trial (Loprinzi, et al., 2000).

  Side effects increase with increasing the dose of venlafaxine from 37.5 mg to 75 mg to 150 mg/day.

  Improvement in other symptoms, such as decreased tiredness and decreased sweating, may occur.

- Clonidine is an alpha-adrenergic agonist used for the relief of hot flashes but can be associated with significant side effects such as dry mouth, constipation, itching, and drowsiness.

  Low-dose clonidine (0.1 mg/day), administered either in pill form or by a transdermal patch, reduces the frequency and severity of vasomotor symptoms.

  Dose escalation is associated with improved response.

  Side effects of dizziness, nausea, dry mouth, and headache make higher doses unacceptable for some women.

- Bellergal (ergotamine tartrate), belladonna alkaloids, and phenobarbital have been used to treat hot flashes.

However, potential addictive risk and the availability of safer alternatives limit the usefulness of these agents.

- Low-dose progestational agents have demonstrated some efficacy but are also associated with significant side effects.

  Medroxyprogesterone acetate (Provera)

  Megestrol acetate 20 mg (Megace)

  Are associated with menstrual bleeding

  Other side effects: breast tenderness, mood changes, and abdominal bloating, which may affect acceptability and adherence

- Vitamin E (Barton, et al., 1998)

  Used for many years to treat hot flashes in healthy women. However, vitamin E has extremely limited effectiveness, if any, in decreasing hot flashes in women with breast cancer.

  Recommended doses vary but are in the range of 200 to 800 IU QID.

  Women with heart disease, diabetes, or hypertension must consult their physicians before taking vitamin E.

Nonpharmacologic Management of Hot Flashes

- Behavioral strategies
  1. Relaxation training, such as progressive muscle relaxation, may decrease sympathetic nervous system arousal.

2. Dietary changes, with avoidance of caffeine and alcohol, are recommended but these dietary changes have not been empirically tested.

3. Phytoestrogen intake through either soy-based or botanical products has been recommended for reducing hot flashes. However, several study results are conflicting and the definitive benefits of soy in relieving hot flashes are unclear and the effects of long-term use of soy products in breast cancer survivors are unknown.

4. Regular physical exercise is also recommended, but empirical studies are needed to confirm the benefit of physical exercise in reducing hot flashes.

5. Acupuncture is being evaluated in clinical trials as an intervention for relief for hot flashes.

6. Herbal remedies and vitamins have limited effectiveness (Hunter, et al., 2004).

Skeletal Effects: Osteoporosis (Mahon, 1998)

- Reduction in bone mass, leading to osteoporosis and bone fracture.
- There is low bone mass with microarchitectural deterioration.
- The normal bone modeling consists of bone resorption and bone formation.

  Osteoblasts are cells that facilitate bone formation.

  Osteoclasts are cells that facilitate bone resorption.

> *When osteoclast activity is not replenished by osteoblast activity, there is a net decrease in the total bone formation leading to a decrease in bone mass.*

- Women with osteoporosis are at increased risk of osteoporotic fractures of the distal forearm, spine, and hip.
- Women with breast cancer are at higher risk of osteoporosis than the general population of aging women for several reasons:
  1. Women who receive chemotherapy experience premature menopause at an earlier age and with lower bone mineral density (BMD), compared with women not receiving chemotherapy (Headley, et al., 1998).
  2. Breast cancer survivors are not candidates for HRT and may lose up to 30% of bone mass within the first year of menopause without estrogen.
- Other risk factors for osteoporosis

  Advancing age.

  Family history of osteoporosis.

  Ethnicity: Caucasian and Asian women have higher risks and African-American and Hispanic women have lower risks.

  Small body size and low body weight (less than 127 pounds).

- Diagnosis of osteoporosis

  Bone mineral density studies, DEXA scan, repeated every 2 years.

- Pharmacologic management

  Calcitonin is indicated for treatment of osteoporosis only. Calcitonin is a naturally occurring hormone that is involved in calcium regulation and reduces bone loss in the spine.

  Estrogen/hormone replacement therapy is used to prevent and to treat osteoporosis but is generally contraindicated in women with breast cancer.

  Bisphosphonates reduce bone loss by inhibiting the action of osteoclasts and reduce vertebral fractures (Delmas, et al., 1997).

  Alendronate and risedronate are approved for the treatment of osteoporosis.

  Selective estrogen receptor modulators (SERMs) such as raloxifene may augment BMD.

- Nonpharmacologic interventions (Mahon, 1998; Slemenda & Johnston Jr., 1999)

  Nonpharmacologic interventions are also very important interventions used to treat osteoporosis.

  Exercise 30 minutes a day, three times a week.

  Adhere to a weight-bearing, strength, and weight-training program that is frequent and progressive in intensity.

  Improve environment to reduce the risk of falls (wear sturdy, low-heeled shoes; secure rugs in home).

- Nutritional changes

  High-calcium diet, including dairy products (i.e., milk, yogurt, ice cream, cheese), fruits, vegetables (e.g., broccoli, legumes, kale), and tofu (i.e., soy, soy milk).

Calcium supplements of 1,500 mg/day in divided doses of 500 mg, with vitamin D 200 to 400 IU to help absorb calcium.

Do not take calcium supplements with caffeine, which can affect the absorption of calcium.

Stop smoking and decrease alcohol intake.

- Web site resources

  National Osteoporosis Foundation (NOF) is a nonprofit, voluntary health organization dedicated to reducing the prevalence of osteoporosis. NOF can be accessed online at www.nof.org.

Cardiovascular Effects

- Cardiovascular disease is the leading cause of death in women in the United States.

- Risk of cardiovascular disease increases with estrogen deficiency.

- Estrogen has a protective cardiovascular effect. When estrogen is decreased, it causes changes in the plasma total cholesterol and lipid profile.

- Decreased estrogen results in a higher level of low-density lipoprotein (LDL) cholesterol and a lower concentration of high-density lipoprotein (HDL) cholesterol.

- Other risk factors for cardiovascular disease include obesity, hypertension, diabetes, sedentary lifestyle, and cigarette smoking.

- The evaluation of the incidence of cardiovascular disease in breast cancer survivors represents an important and growing area of research.

- There is controversy in the potential protective effect of estrogen replacement therapy on cardiovascular risk. Findings from the Women's Health Initiative study indicate an increased risk of cardiovascular disease, stroke, and pulmonary embolism in women who took combined conjugated equine estrogen and medroxyprogesterone acetate.

- Table 17-1 lists management strategies to reduce the risk of cardiovascular disease.

Urogenital Tract (Goodman, 1999)

- The vagina and urethra have active estrogen receptor sites in the epithelium. With menopause, there is resulting changes in the urogenital tract.

- Atrophic changes in the vagina result in vaginal dryness, dyspareunia, and atrophic vaginitis.

- Urogenital atrophy and urinary symptoms include dysuria, frequency, urgency, nocturia, urinary stress incontinence, and urinary tract infections.

- Decrease in vaginal lubrication, atrophic vaginitis, and frequent infection can result in dyspareunia.

- Changes in the urogenital tract are bothersome and can impair one's quality of life.

- Management:

  Water-soluble lubricants have been the historical intervention when estrogen (systemic or cream) is contraindicated.

  Vaginal lubricants include KY jelly, Replens, and Astroglide

  Replens has been reported to increase vaginal moisture and elasticity and return vaginal pH to its pre-menopausal state.

  Topical estrogen creams and tablets are also used to treat vaginal dryness.

TABLE 17-1
Management Strategies to Reduce Cardiovascular Disease Risk

- Stop smoking.
- Exercise 30 minutes a day, three times a week.
- Eat a moderate diet to lower fat intake and control blood lipid levels.
- Take vitamin E, 400 to 800 units, which has a protective effect against coronary artery disease.
- Take dietary supplements of folate plus vitamin B6 and B12, which reduces homocysteine levels and may decrease the risk for CAD.
- Take aspirin, 75 to 325 mg per day, which offers protection against CAD.
- Prescribe lipid- and cholesterol-modifying medications for patients with an unfavorable profile.
- Maintain a healthy body weight.

Source: Data from Castelli, 2000; Goodman, 1996; Gorodeski & Utian, 1994.

- Management of urinary symptoms:

  Many pharmacologic interventions can be used to treat urge incontinence.

  Smooth muscle relaxants such as hyoscyamine and oxybutynin have been used for urge incontinence.

  Other drugs used to treat urge incontinence include antihistamines and tricyclic antidepressants.

  Estrogen to treat urinary incontinence is questionable.

  Few pharmacologic interventions are available to treat stress incontinence. These include alpha-adrenergic agonists such as pseudoephedrine, ephedrine, and phenylpropanolamine to stimulate the smooth muscle of the bladder anatomy.

  Behavioral interventions include:

  1. Kegel strengthening exercises
  2. Bladder training program
  3. Void at regular time intervals
  4. Promote adequate fluid intake

Recommendations for Nursing Practice

- Implications for practice are related to assessment, patient education, symptom management, monitoring of treatment outcomes, and clinical research.
- Assessment of a multisystem profile of demographic factors, breast cancer and treatment-related factors, extent of physical effects of menopausal symptoms.

- Educate women and their family members about the possibility of menopausal symptoms, risk factors, and potential impact on quality of life.

- Management using both pharmacologic and non-pharmacologic strategies and the effectiveness of complementary and alternative therapies.

- Promote health-improving routines such as exercise and nutritional changes.

- Multidisciplinary management adds benefit.

REFERENCES

Barton, D. L., Loprinzi, C. L., Quella, S. K., Sloan, J. A., Veeder, M. H., Egner, J. R., et al. (1998). Prospective evaluation of vitamin E for hot flashes in breast cancer survivors. *Journal of Clinical Oncology, 16*(2), 495–500.

Carpenter, J. (February, 2001). *Hot flashes and other menopausal symptoms in breast cancer survivors and age-matched healthy comparison women.* Paper presented at the Sixth National Conference on Cancer Nursing Research Oncology Nursing Society, Jacksonville, FL.

Carpenter, J., & Elam, J. (2004). Menopausal symptoms. In K. H. Dow (Ed.), *Contemporary issues in breast cancer: A nursing persective* (2nd ed., pp. 230–262). Sudbury, MA: Jones & Bartlett.

Carpenter, J. S. (2000). Hot flashes and their management in breast cancer. *Seminars in Oncology Nursing, 16*(3), 214–225.

Castelli, W. P. (2000). Menopause and cardiovascular disease. In B. A. Eskin (Ed.), *The menopause: comprehensive management, 4th ed.*, pp. 1117–1135. New York: Parthenon.

Cobleigh, M. (2000). Managing menopausal problems. In J. R. Harris, M. Lippman, M. Morrow & C. K. Osborne (Eds.), *Diseases of the breast* (2nd ed., pp. 1041–1050). Philadelphia: Lippincott Williams & Wilkins.

Delmas, P. D., Balena, R., Confravreux, E., Hardouin, C., Hardy, P., & Bremond, A. (1997). Bisphosphonate risedronate prevents bone loss in women with artificial menopause due to chemotherapy of breast cancer: A double-blind, placebo-controlled study. *Journal of Clinical Oncology, 15*(3), 955–962.

Freedman, R. R. (1998). Biochemical, metabolic, and vascular mechanisms in menopausal hot flashes. *Fertility and Sterility, 74*, 332–337.

Freedman, R. R., & Krell, W. (1999). Reduced thermoregulatory null zone in postmenopausal women with hot flashes. *American Journal of Obstetrics and Gynecology, 181*, 66–70.

Goodman, M. (1996). Menopausal symptoms. In C. H. Yarbro, M. H. Frogge, & M. Goodman (Eds.), *Cancer symptom management*, pp. 77–99. Sudbury, Mass.: Jones & Bartlett.

Goodman, M. (1999). Menopausal symptoms. In C. H. Yarbro, M. H. Frogge, & M. Goodman (Eds.), *Cancer symptom management* (2nd ed., pp. 95–111). Sudbury, MA: Jones & Bartlett.

Gorodeski, G. I., & Utian, W. H. (1994). Epidemiology of risk factors of cardiovascular disease in postmenopausal women. In R. A. Lobo (Ed.), *Treatment of the postmenopausal woman: Basic and clinical aspects*, pp. 199–221. New York: Raven Press.

Headley, J. A., Theriault, R. L., LeBlanc, A. D., Vassilopoulou-Sellin, R., & Hortobagyi, G. N. (1998). Pilot study of bone mineral density in breast cancer patients treated with adjuvant chemotherapy. *Cancer Investigation, 16*(1), 6–11.

Hunter, M. S., Grunfeld, E. A., Mittal, S., Sikka, P., Ramirez, A. J., Fentiman, I., et al. (2004). Menopausal symptoms in women with breast cancer: Prevalence and treatment preferences. *Psychooncology, 13*(11), 769–778.

Loprinzi, C. L., Kugler, J. W., Sloan, J. A., Mailliard, J. A., LaVasseur, B. I., Barton, D. L., et al. (2000). Venlafaxine in management of hot flashes in survivors of breast cancer: A randomised controlled trial. *Lancet, 356*(9247), 2059–2063.

Mahon, S. M. (1998). Osteoporosis: A concern for cancer survivors. *Oncology Nursing Forum, 25*(5), 843–851.

Slemenda, C. W., & Johnston Jr., C. C. (1999). Epidemiology of osteoporosis. In R. A. Lobo (Ed.), *Treatment of the postmenopausal women: Basic and clinical aspects* (2nd ed., pp. 279–285). Philadelphia: Lippincott Williams & Wilkins.

Snyder, G. M., Sielsch, E. C., & Reville, B. (1998). The controversy of hormone-replacement therapy in breast cancer survivors. *Oncology Nursing Forum, 25*(4), 699–706.

Swain, S., Santen, R., Burger, H., & Pritchard, K. (1999). Treatment of estrogen deficiency symptoms in women surviving breast cancer. Part 4: Urogenital atrophy, vasomotor instability, sleep disorders, and related symptoms. *Oncology, 13*, 551–575.

Utian, W. H. (2001). Semantics, menopause-related terminology, and the straw reproductive aging staging system. *Menopause, 8*(6), 398–401.

CHAPTER EIGHTEEN

Reproductive Effects

Overview (Dow & Kuhn, 2004)

- Although the incidence of breast cancer in pre-menopausal women is less than 20%, the impact of treatment on fertility is a major distress and a significant quality-of-life concern.

- At the time of breast cancer diagnosis, young women may either be planning or starting to have a family. The diagnosis and treatment of breast cancer interrupt these plans.

- There are many factors that have an effect on fertility and reproduction. These include treatment factors such as chemotherapy and hormonal therapy and personal factors such as age, previous reproductive history, weight, and smoking history.

- Advancing age and alkylating agents are known risk factors that can affect fertility.

- The addition of taxanes in adjuvant chemotherapy and tamoxifen have increased overall length of treatment, thus rendering women at increased risk of infertility.

- Assisted reproductive technologies (ARTs) have helped changed fertility and pregnancy outcomes in younger women with breast cancer.

Impact of Breast Cancer Treatment on Fertility

- Breast cancer treatment can have a variable effect on fertility.

- Mastectomy alone does not affect one's fertility, but influences the future ability of the woman to breast-feed from the affected side.

- Radiation therapy

    Contraindicated during pregnancy

    After treatment may influence ability to breast-feed from irradiated breast

- Chemotherapy (Hensley & Reichman, 1998; Meirow, 2000; Moore, 2000; Minton & Munster, 2002)

    Small fraction of ovarian follicles cycle during any one time, with the cycling cells most susceptible to damage from chemotherapy.

    Cyclophosphamide-containing adjuvant therapy results in endocrine hormone profiles that are consistent with primary ovarian failure:

    1. Fall in estradiol and progesterone levels

2.   Elevation in follicle-stimulating hormone (FSH) and luteinizing hormone (LH) levels

3.   Increase in vaginal epithelial atrophy and endometrial hypoplasia

Degree of amenorrhea is variable and is related to dose regimens and total dose of cyclophosphamide.

Temporary amenorrhea occurs more often in younger women because they have a larger ovarian reserve.

Permanent amenorrhea occurs when there is complete destruction of ovarian follicles.

Doxorubicin does not appreciably increase the risk of amenorrhea when added to cyclophosphamide.

Onset of amenorrhea is age related, with decreased likelihood of regaining menses after age 45 after adjuvant chemotherapy.

Anthracycline-based chemotherapy (AC) combination (doxorubicin + cyclophosphamide) has less ovarian toxicity than cyclophosphamide, methotrexate, fluorouracil (CMF)-based chemotherapy.

- Tamoxifen (Ibrahim, et al., 2003)

  Use results in an increase in estradiol and total estrogen levels without a significant rise in FSH or LH.

  Even when women do not experience amenorrhea with tamoxifen, they are on hormonal therapy for at least 5 years and cannot attempt pregnancy during tamoxifen treatment.

  Women can get pregnant while on tamoxifen therapy and thus should use appropriate contraception.

> *Women should wait until 2 months after tamoxifen therapy has ended before attempting pregnancy, due to the long half-life of tamoxifen.*

- Taxane therapy

  The risk of amenorrhea with addition of taxanes in adjuvant chemotherapy on ovarian function is considered small.

- Bone marrow transplantation (BMT)

  BMT is associated with a high rate of ovarian failure, and women who receive high-dose chemotherapy should expect permanent amenorrhea.

Personal Factors that Influence Amenorrhea

- A healthy 30-year-old woman has a 20% chance each month of getting pregnant compared to a healthy 40-year-old woman having a 5% chance of getting pregnant (American Society for Reproductive Medicine can be accessed online at www.asrm.org).

- Fertility rates decline significantly after age 40 in the normal population without breast cancer.

- Advancing age in combination with cyclophosphamide has an effect on development of amenorrhea (Koyama, et al., 1977).

  Average cumulative dose of 5.2 g cyclophosphamide has resulted in amenorrhea among women in their 40s, compared with 9.3 g cyclophosphamide among women in their 30s.

CMF: Amenorrhea in women age 40 years was 40%, compared with 76% in women over the age of 40 (Bines, et al., 1996).

AC: No incidence of amenorrhea at 1 year after AC in women younger than age 45 years, compared with women over age 45 years.

- Being overweight (with a body mass index between 25–29) and obesity (BMI >30) has a negative impact on fertility.

  Overweight and obese women tend to have irregular or infrequent menstrual cycles.

  Women with history of breast cancer may have unwanted weight gain of up to 20% over normal weight after adjuvant chemotherapy.

  Thus, there is an increased risk of amenorrhea.

- Smoking contributes to infertility and decreases a woman's chances of carrying a pregnancy to term.

  Smoking accelerates the loss of eggs and decreases reproductive function.

  When women stop smoking, they improve their chance of becoming pregnant and carrying the pregnancy to term.

Effects of Subsequent Pregnancy on Survival

- There have been no epidemiologic studies, to date, that have suggested an adverse effect of pregnancy on survival.

- Results of retrospective institutional reports between 1940 and 1979, case-control studies between 1965 and 1997, and population-based studies (1994 to 1999) have not shown an adverse effect on survival.

- Potential form of bias called "healthy mother effect" may explain why women who become pregnant may be more likely to be free of the disease at the time of pregnancy, compared with women who do not have subsequent pregnancy (Sankila, et al., 1994).

- Hormonal changes that occur during pregnancy have shown little influence on recurrence (Gelber, et al., 2001).

- Some studies suggest equal or improved survival in multiple pregnancies.

Risk of Spontaneous Abortion After Breast Cancer

- Rate of miscarriage was 24% among 53 women with breast cancer who became pregnant after diagnosis, compared with 18% in 265 case-matched control subjects who never had breast cancer (Velentgas, et al., 1999).

Fertility Options Before and After Treatment
(Oktay, et al., 2003; Dow, 2004; Dow & Kuhn, 2004)

- Ideally, it is best for young women to understand their fertility options before adjuvant chemotherapy begins.

- It is also important for young women to understand that despite their best attempts, they may not be able to preserve their fertility.

- First suggestion is to discuss chemotherapy options with their medical oncologist. A chemotherapy regimen that contains smaller total dose of cyclophosphamide may be considered.

- Consider an evaluation by a reproductive endocrinologist before treatment begins. Several options using assisted reproductive technology (ART) may be discussed.

- Ovarian suppression using a gonadotropin-releasing hormone (GnRH) agonist has been used to reduce ovarian toxicity in other young cancer survivors, but its effect in preserving fertility in young women with breast cancer has been small (Blumenfeld, et al., 1996).

- Options after treatment may include consideration of adoption or child-free living.

Questions/Concerns About Pregnancy After Breast Cancer

- What is a reasonable amount of time to wait before attempting a pregnancy?

  Each woman must feel psychologically and physically in shape after cancer treatment before starting a pregnancy.

  Suggestions from the literature are variable, with most suggesting a wait of at least 1 year.

  Other suggestions from the literature recommend at least a 2-year wait, until the greatest risk of recurrence has passed. However, risk of recurrence can be up to 25 years after treatment.

Other quality-of-life considerations must be taken into account. For example, younger women who receive adjuvant chemotherapy and continue to menstruate are at higher risk for early menopause. If young women desire pregnancy, they need to consider pregnancy sooner rather than later, with reduced chances of conception.

- Will more than one pregnancy affect recurrence?

  Limited data do not indicate that more than one pregnancy adversely influences recurrence.

- What is the safety in breast-feeding?

  If a woman has received breast-conserving surgery and radiation therapy, there will be either diminished or absent milk production in the irradiated breast.

  Radiation causes ductal shrinkage, condensation of cytoplasm lining the duct, atrophy of lobules, and perilobar and periductal fibrosis

- What is the health of children of women with breast cancer?

  Evidence does not suggest an adverse effect on the health of infants born to mothers with a history of breast cancer.

- What circumstances may occur to suggest termination of pregnancy?

  There are no easy answers, and there must be a highly individualized discussion.

  In situations in which a patient develops recurrence/metastatic disease during the first trimester of pregnancy and must start adjuvant chemotherapy and/or radiation therapy, discussion of pregnancy termination is necessary.

Adoption as an Alternative to Pregnancy

- Women must come to terms with amenorrhea and infertility after breast cancer treatment.
- Support is needed from the oncology team, spouse/significant other, and family.
- Women must have the financial means to go through an adoption.
- Process of adoption may take up to several years.

Nursing Issues

- Initiate discussions about the potential for amenorrhea earlier in the diagnostic and treatment phase rather than later in the survivorship experience.
- Discussions must occur over time and with a supportive oncology team.
- Amenorrhea is variable, depending on adjuvant chemotherapy dose of cyclophosphamide and patient age.
- There is no epidemiologic, clinical, or prognostic evidence that pregnancy or its termination will alter the natural history of breast or other cancers.
- Treatment has little influence on the health of the offspring.

REFERENCES

American Society for Reproductive Medicine. (2004). Retrieved February 22, 2005, from www.asrm.org

Bines, J., Oleske, D., & Cobleigh, M. (1996). Ovarian function in premenopausal women treated with adjuvant therapy for breast cancer. *Journal of Clinical Oncology, 14,* 1718–1729.

Blumenfeld, Z., Avivi, I., Linn, S., Epelbaum, R., Ben-Shahar, M., & Haim, N. (1996). Prevention of irreversible chemotherapy-induced ovarian damage in young women with lymphoma by a gonadotrophin-releasing hormone agonist in parallel to chemotherapy. *Human Reproduction, 11,* 1620–1626.

Dow, K. H. (2004). Psychosocial issues of fertility preservation in cancer survivors. In T. Tulandi & R. G. Gosden (Eds.), *Preservation of fertility* (pp. 237–246). London: Taylor & Francis.

Dow, K. H., & Kuhn, D. (2004). Fertility options in young breast cancer survivors: A review of the literature. *Oncology Nursing Forum, 31*(3), E46–E53.

Gelber, S., Coates, A. S., Goldhrsch, A., Castiglione-Gertsch, M., Marini, G., Lindtner, J., et al. (2001). Effects of pregnancy on overall survival after the diagnosis of early-stage breast cancer. *Journal of Clinical Oncology, 19,* 1671–1675.

Hensley, M. L., & Reichman, B. S. (1998). Fertility and pregnancy after adjuvant chemotherapy for breast cancer. *Critical Reviews in Oncology and Hematology, 28*(2), 121–128.

Ibrahim, N. K., Machneil, S., Headley, J. A., Bisotooni, K. T., Buzdar, A. U., & Hortobagyi, G. N. (2003). *Effect of paclitaxel (P)-based chemotherapy on the ovarian failure (OF) of breast cancer patients (pts): A retrospective study.* Paper presented at the ASCO American Society of Clinical Oncology, Chicago, IL.

Koyama, H., Wada, T., Nishizawa, Y., Iwanaga, T., & Aoki, Y. (1977). Cyclophosphamide-induced ovarian failure and its therapeutic significance in patients with breast cancer. *Cancer, 39*(4), 1403–1409.

Meirow, D. (2000). Reproduction post-chemotherapy in young cancer patients. *Molecular and Cellular Endocrinology, 169*(1–2), 123–131.

Minton, S. E., & Munster, P. N. (2002). Chemotherapy-induced amenorrhea and fertility in women undergoing adjuvant treatment for breast cancer. *Cancer Control, 9*(6), 466–472.

Moore, H. (2000). Fertility and the impact of systemic therapy on hormonal status following treatment for breast cancer. *Current Oncology Reports, 2*, 587–593.

Oktay, K., Buyuk, E., Davis, O., Yermakova, I., Veeck, L., & Rosenwaks, Z. (2003). Fertility preservation in breast cancer patients: IVF and embryo cryopreservation after ovarian stimulation with tamoxifen. *Human Reproduction, 18*(1), 90–95.

Sankila, R., Heinavaara, S., & Hakulinen, T. (1994). Survival of breast cancer patients after subsequent term pregnancy: "Healthy mother effect." *American Journal of Obstetrics and Gynecology, 170*(3), 818–823.

Velentgas, P., Daling, J. R., Malone, K. E., Weiss, N. S., Williams, M. A., Self, S. G., et al. (1999). Pregnancy after breast carcinoma: Outcomes and influence on mortality. *Cancer, 85*, 2301–2305, 2424–2432.

CHAPTER NINETEEN

Late Physical Effects of Cancer Treatment

Overview (Loerzel, 2004)

- Major advances in breast cancer treatment have increased survival so that women can live cancer free for many years.

- Unfortunately, late effects of therapy can have a lasting impact on health and the quality of life.

- Late physical effects of cancer treatment are a growing concern among breast cancer survivors.

- This chapter reviews late effects that occur several months to many years after treatment has ended.

- Late effects include major organ toxicity to the heart and lungs, cognitive dysfunction, neurosensory changes, skeletal changes, and secondary cancers.

Late Cardiac Effects (Loerzel, 2004; Loerzel & Dow, 2003)

- Cardiac dysfunction can result from radiation therapy to the left breast, doxorubicin doses greater than 550 mg/m^2, combination chemotherapy with doxorubicin and radiation therapy to the left breast or chest, and treatment with trastuzumab.

- Advancing age and preexisting cardiac disease are additional factors that increase cardiac injury.

- Older radiation therapy techniques, with higher radiation dose to the heart, resulted in late cardiac effects.

- Chemotherapeutic agents that can lead to serious cardiac complications include doxorubicin and trastuzumab.

  1. Doxorubicin

     Damage may be related to free radical release during treatment leading to cell damage in the myocardium.

     Cardiac abnormalities include EKC changes, congestive heart failure (CHF), and cardiomyopathy.

     Factors that increase the risk of cardiac damage include advancing age, preexisting cardiac disease or hypertension, concomitant cyclophosphamide, and sequential trastuzumab therapy.

     Incidence of CHF in patients with doxorubicin-based chemotherapy varies based on total cumulative dose.

Standard four cycles of doxorubicin (A) and cyclophosphamide (C) with maximum total dose of doxorubicin 450 mg/m^2 is generally not associated with an increase in CHF.

When total cumulative dose of doxorubicin is less than 500–550 mg/m^2, incidence of cardiomyopathy declines.

a. Cyclophosphamide

Cyclophosphamide is not associated with cardiotoxicity when given alone at standard doses.

Cardiotoxicity increases when this agent is combined with doxorubicin.

b. Taxanes

Taxanes are not associated with cardiotoxicity when given alone at standard doses.

Cardiotoxicity increases in some patients when these agents are combined with doxorubicin.

2. Trastuzumab

Trastuzumab alone can have a direct effect on the myocardium, but its cardiac effect is synergistic when combined with doxorubicin.

Cardiac damage may be expressed as a decrease in ejection fraction, cardiomyopathy, and CHF.

• Radiation pericarditis

Pericarditis is a late effect of radiation to the left chest and heart.

Pericarditis is a rare late radiation effect and is associated with the volume of heart in the radiation treatment field, dose fractionation, and total radiation dose.

It is known that pericardial and myocardial cells are sensitive to radiation damage, causing edema and rupture of capillaries leading to fibrosis.

Fortunately, today, advances in radiation therapy techniques either prevent or limit the amount of radiation to the left chest and heart muscle.

- Cardiac symptoms

Cardiac symptoms vary depending on the type and degree of damage.

Early symptoms include increased fatigue, decreased ability to engage in exercise, palpitations, and shortness of breath.

Early cardiac symptoms may be attributed to menopausal changes.

In addition, women may not complain of chest pain. Rather, they may describe symptoms of "heaviness in the chest" or attribute the problem to fatigue.

Severe and late symptoms include dyspnea at rest, tachycardia, diaphoresis, and hypotension. Even with late symptoms, women may not complain of chest pain.

Thus, careful cardiac assessment is needed during the follow-up exam.

- Prevention and management of cardiac dysfunction

  Preventing cardiotoxicity during treatment include lowering total cumulative dose of doxorubicin, evaluation of preexisting cardiac and peripheral vascular disease prior to treatment, increased monitoring of patients on trastuzumab, and the use of cardioprotectants. In addition, newer radiation therapy techniques can either prevent or limit the amount of radiation to the left chest and heart.

  Management of cardiac dysfunction includes early referral to a cardiologist for evaluation. Cardiac work-up may include standard EKG, blood studies, cardiac stress test, echocardiogram, and cardiac catheterization. Treatments vary depending on the degree of cardiac damage and may include diuretics, beta blockers, calcium channel blockers, and digoxin.

Late Pulmonary Effects (Loerzel, 2004)

- Chemotherapy and radiation therapy can have late adverse effects on the lungs.
- Chemotherapeutic agents that may increase risk of late pulmonary effects include high-dose cyclophosphamide, methotrexate, doxorubicin, and taxanes.

  Pulmonary late effects include pneumonitis and fibrosis that can occur several months to years after treatment.

These late effects were more common when high-dose chemotherapy was used rather than standard doses of chemotherapy.

- Radiation pneumonitis

  Radiation pneumonitis is related to the total volume of lung tissue radiated, dose fractionation, and total radiation dose.

  Patients at risk include those receiving radiation to the supraclavicular and axillary nodal regions and three-field rather than two-field radiation treatment.

  Pneumonitis occurs in 1% of patients about 6 to 18 months after radiation ends.

  Generally, this late effect occurs in patients having more than 10% lung volume treated.

  Symptoms are generally transient and include dry non-productive cough, low grade fever, shortness of breath, and fullness in the chest.

  Careful assessment and follow-up is needed because symptoms of radiation pneumonitis are similar to pulmonary metastasis.

- Radiation fibrosis

  Radiation fibrosis is a late effect that can occur several months to years after treatment.

  Radiation fibrosis may naturally progress from radiation pneumonitis or may occur independently.

  Early symptoms include shortness of breath, decreased ability to exercise, and orthopnea.

Late and severe symptoms include cyanosis, chronic cor pulmonale, and finger clubbing.

Treatment is aimed at symptomatic relief with prednisone and supportive care.

Thus, prevention of radiation fibrosis is the key with newer radiation techniques that limit the amount of total lung volume.

Cognitive Deficits (Loerzel, 2004; Tannock, et al., 2004; O'Shaughnessy, 2003; Wefel, et al., 2004)

- Impaired cognitive deficits, as a late effect of breast cancer treatment, have received increased attention in recent years.

- Women have reported problems with concentration, short-term memory loss, decreased attention span, and difficulty with problem solving.

- Cognitive deficits are subtle and can interfere with the quality of life.

- Most often, these cognitive deficits were previously attributed to either advancing age and/or menopausal symptoms.

- Cognitive dysfunction is most often related to high-dose chemotherapy. It is often called *chemobrain*.

- However, cognitive dysfunction can precede chemotherapy in women with nonmetastatic disease. Hormone replacement therapy and current menopausal status must be taken into account before attributing cognitive dysfunction entirely to chemotherapy.

- Treatment

  Recombinant human endogenous erythropoietin (epoetin alfa) is an established treatment for chemotherapy-related anemia and has been evaluated as a potential neuroprotective agent to reduce cognitive deficits.

- Cognitive deficits are a growing concern among breast cancer survivors. Thus, recommendations for future research to evaluate cognitive deficits include the following:

  Evaluate the discrepancies between subject complaints of cognitive dysfunction and objective measures of cognitive testing.

  Prospectively compare the presence of cognitive deficits, contributing factors, and underlying mechanisms in patients with deficits and those without deficit.

  Examine cognitive deficits in patients with cancers other than breast cancer.

  Develop animal models and imaging techniques to better understand underlying mechanism of cognitive dysfunction.

Neurosensory Deficits

- Late neurosensory deficits can occur as a result of high-dose chemotherapy, treatment with paclitaxel, and radiation therapy.

- Peripheral neuropathy is a known acute side effect of paclitaxel. Dose-sense long-term weekly infusions of paclitaxel increase the risk of peripheral neuropathy (Lombardi, et al., 2004).

- Brachial plexopathy is a rare late effect of radiation therapy. It occurs more often when patients received axillary radiation causing fibrosis to the axilla and supraclavicular regions (Bajrovic, et al., 2004). This injury is radiation dose related and rarely occurs with doses less than 50 Gy delivered over 5 weeks (e.g., 56 Gy in 15 fractions to the axilla have higher risk of brachial plexopathy).

- Signs and aymptoms of brachial plexopathy:
    1. Mild discomfort in the shoulder and arm
    2. Paresthesias and weakness in the arm and hand that are progressive
    3. Evidence of soft-tissue fibrosis in supraclavicular and infraclavicular regions

- Prevention and management

    Careful assessment is needed because it is difficult clinically to differentiate brachial plexopathy from recurrence.

    There is no recognized treatment for brachial plexopathy. Thus, prevention is key.

- Reversible brachial plexopathy occurs at radiation doses less than 50 Gy and has a short latency period, with a median of about 4.5 months.

- Soft-tissue necrosis is associated with postoperative XRT.

    This late effect rarely occurs today with modern radiation techniques and dose fractionation.

> *Incidence increases with higher radiation dose or changes in fractionation schedules.*
>
> *Patients older than 60 years are at higher risk.*

Skeletal Changes

- Rib fractures are associated with radiation therapy.
- Rib fractures occur in the radiated field in about 1% of patients.
- The median time to occurrence of this late effect is about 12 months.
- Rib fractures occur more often in patients treated with 4-meV (million electron volt) radiation treatment machines, compared with 6-meV or 8-meV treatment machines and are most likely related to increased radiation dose to the lateral rib cage.
- Other risk factors for rib fractures include:
  1. Prior trauma to the area
  2. Adjuvant chemotherapy
- Rib fracture does not necessarily represent bony metastases.
- Rib fractures are generally asymptomatic or associated with mild discomfort.
- Treatment includes nonnarcotic analgesics and anti-inflammatory agents.
- Osteoporotic changes that occur with treatment are discussed in Chapter 17.

Secondary Cancers

- Breast cancer survivors are at an increased risk of developing breast cancer in the ipsilateral breast.

- In addition, breast cancer survivors with an inherited predisposition are at an increased risk of developing ovarian cancer.

- Secondary cancers are a late effect resulting from chemotherapy and radiation therapy.

- High-dose chemotherapy with yclophosphamide increases the risk of developing myeloproliferative disease and acute leukemia.

- Radiation therapy may contribute to the development of contralateral breast cancer and sarcoma.

    Latency period between exposure and detection is about 10 years.

    Risk of carcinogenesis increases with doses up to 10 Gy and then levels off and declines.

    Radiation dose to the opposite, unaffected breast is about 1 to 3 Gy and, thus, tumor induction in the ipsilateral breast may occur.

    Risk also increases when radiation is given at a younger age (less than 40 years).

- Soft-tissue sarcoma

    Soft-tissue sarcoma is a rare complication that occurred in patients having had a mastectomy and postoperative XRT.

    Fortunately, with advanced radiation techniques used today, this late effect is very rare.

REFERENCES

Bajrovic, A., Rades, D., Fehlauer, F., Tribius, S., Hoeller, U., Rudat, V., et al. (2004). Is there a life-long risk of brachial plexopathy after radiotherapy of supraclavicular lymph nodes in breast cancer patients? *Radiotherapy and Oncology, 71*(3), 297–301.

Loerzel, V. W. (2004). Late physical effects of cancer treatment. In K. H. Dow (Ed.), *Contemporary issues in breast cancer: A nursing persective* (2nd ed., pp. 263–280). Sudbury, MA: Jones & Bartlett.

Loerzel, V. W., & Dow, K. H. (2003). Cardiac toxicity related to cancer treatment. *Clinical Journal of Oncology Nursing, 7*(5), 557–562.

Lombardi, D., Crivellari, D., Scuderi, C., Magri, M. D., Spazzapan, S., Sorio, R., et al. (2004). Long-term, weekly 1-hour infusion of paclitaxel in patients with metastatic breast cancer: A phase II monoinstitutional study. *Tumori, 90*(3), 285–288.

O'Shaughnessy, J. A. (2003). Chemotherapy-induced cognitive dysfunction: A clearer picture. *Clinical Breast Cancer,* (4 Suppl 2), S89–94.

Tannock, I. F., Ahles, T. A., Ganz, P. A., & Van Dam, F. S. (2004). Cognitive impairment associated with chemotherapy for cancer: Report of a workshop. *Journal of Clinical Oncology, 22*(11), 2233–2239.

Wefel, J. S., Lenzi, R., Theriault, R., Buzdar, A. U., Cruickshank, S., & Meyers, C. A. (2004). "Chemobrain" in breast carcinoma?: A prologue. *Cancer, 101*(3), 466–475.

CHAPTER TWENTY

Survivorship Issues

Background

- *Quality of life* (QOL) is a term referring to a general sense of well-being, encompassing a multidimensional perspective including physical, psychological, social, and spiritual well-being (Dow, et al., 1996).

- *Survivorship* definition is based on the National Coalition for Cancer Survivorship and is defined as the process of living through and beyond a cancer diagnosis (Clark, et al., 1996).

- Breast cancer survivors include those newly diagnosed, regardless of the stage of disease; those actively receiving treatment; those having recurrence, secondary cancers, and metastatic disease; and long-term survivors without evidence of breast cancer.

- Evidence suggests that multidisciplinary models with strong clinical and advanced-practice nursing make a difference in patient satisfaction and adjustment and improved QOL (Frost, et al., 1999; Ritz, et al., 2000).

- Women with breast cancer face myriad concerns after treatment ends. Many of the physical and psychological complications are described in the literature. Less evident are the social and spiritual well-being concerns.

- Common physical effects during survivorship (See Chapters 15–19 for further discussion of these concerns):

  Lymphedema

  Fatigue and sleep disturbance

  Menopausal symptoms

  Reproductive concerns

- Psychological concerns during survivorship (Bennett, et al., 2004)

  Anxiety

  Depression

  Fear of recurrence and uncertainty over the future

- Social concerns during survivorship

  Family relationships

  Work relationships

- Spiritual concerns during survivorship

  Meaning and purpose in life

Anxiety (Lehto & Cimprich, 1999; Montazeri, et al., 2004)

- Anxiety is a complex and universal life experience and is seen as a biobehavioral response to a stimulus that threatens one's physical, psychological, and social well-being.

- Anxiety response involves a subjective feeling of apprehension and heightened physical arousal.

- There are differences between anxiety as a fluctuating temporary state versus anxiety as an inherent personality trait.

- A cognitive appraisal of the threat and stressor as potentially harmful may also produce anxiety.

- Anxiety may influence attention, learning, and coping.

- Risk factors for anxiety include previous mental health, older age, female gender, unrelieved physical symptoms, and concurrent medication causing anxiety (Gobel, 2000).

- Assessment

  State-trait anxiety inventory (STAI) is most commonly used to measure anxiety in patients with cancer. It consists of two scales that measure the state of anxiety and the trait of anxiety (Spielberger, et al., 1983).

- In breast cancer survivors, specific points along the survivorship continuum may induce anxiety. These time points include the completion of cancer therapy; follow-up testing, procedures, and visits;

change in one's oncology team; development of new breast cancer; development of recurrence and metastases; and changes in physical symptoms over time.

- Interventions

  Social support through groups and individual counseling

  Cognitive-behavioral interventions include preparatory information, cognitive restructuring, relaxation and imagery techniques, music therapy, hypnosis, and biofeedback.

  Educational efforts are directed at paced instruction, multiple learning opportunities through use of booklets, pamphlets, video, audio, and Internet-based information.

  Pharmacologic management using benzodiazepines.

  Complementary therapy (Stephenson, et al., 2000).

Depression (Brandt, 1996; Montazeri, et al., 2004; Love, et al., 2004; Badger, et al., 2004)

- Depression may occur in up to 25% of women with breast cancer.

- Women with advanced breast cancer have experienced higher levels of anxiety and depression (up to 25%), which may be persistent.

- A diagnosis of breast cancer may produce mild depressive symptoms. Women with stable personalities and who have adapted well to previous life crises, usually adapt well to a diagnosis of breast cancer and are able to manage their distress.

- Sadness and grief are normal psychological responses for persons faced with either a threatened or an actual loss.

- Depressive symptoms range from mild to severe, from normal states of sadness to clinical syndromes (such as an adjustment disorder with depressed mood) or a major depression.

- Symptoms of depression are similar to cancer treatment effects such as fatigue, sleep-pattern disturbance, changes in diet, and changes in activities of daily living.

- Signs and symptoms of depression:
  1. Fatigue that persists despite rest
  2. Undifferentiated pain
  3. Sleep disturbances in the form of insomnia or hypersomnia
  4. Anxiety or irritability
  5. Gastrointestinal complaints
  6. Differentiate symptoms of disease and treatment side effects from symptoms of clinical depression

- Characteristics of women at high risk:
  1. Personal or family history of depression, substance abuse, and hypochondriasis
  2. Persistent and frequent somatic, psychosomatic, or pain complaints
  3. History of depression before a diagnosis of breast cancer
  4. Advanced stage of disease at diagnosis

- Clinical evaluation (McDonald, et al., 1999):

    1. Assess patient beliefs about the experience of disease and cancer treatment effects.

    2. Diagnosis is based on clusters of symptoms that persist over time and are associated with distress and dysfunction.

- Management of depression requires a multidisciplinary approach with appropriate individualized assessment and patient referral (see Table 20-1).

Fear of Recurrence and Uncertainty over the Future (Loerzel, 2004)

- Fear of recurrence, second cancers, and metastatic disease has a negative influence on psychological well-being.

- Fear of recurrence may be heightened around follow-up visits and anniversary dates and is manifested by heightened anxiety, depression, mood swings, and hypervigilance about health.

- Fear involving recurrence may revolve around the possibility of death, added treatment, pain, advancing disease, emotional distress, and family suffering (Loerzel, 2004).

- Interventions to help reduce fear of recurrence:

    1. Support groups have helped breast cancer survivors within a caring environment address their fear of recurrence, metastasis, and death.

TABLE 20-1

Interventions for Depression

Mild Depression

Validate sadness as a normal reaction to the diagnosis and at various phases of the illness trajectory.

Provide supportive understanding of the multiple personal and physical losses.

Focus on the grief associated with the patient's loss of health.

Emphasize past strengths, support for previous effective coping strategies, and encouragement to mobilize inner resources.

Assist patients in exploring and identifying their purpose in life, the role of spiritual meaning, and in determining effective coping strategies.

Achieve optimal pain control and symptom management.

Recommend exercise programs and behavioral methods, such as relaxation combined with visual imagery suggesting a peaceful scene of the patient's choice.

Refer the patient to the proper support groups.

Moderate to Severe Depression

Cognitive behavioral therapy managed by a clinical psychologist is aimed at controlling target symptoms.

Psychotherapy interventions can be provided by social workers, psychiatric clinical nurse specialists, and psychologists and psychiatrists with knowledge of the specialty of oncology.

Goals are to maintain a primary focus on the illness and its implications, explore issues that affect the adjustment to illness, and reinforce the patient's past coping strategies.

Pharmacologic therapy may be indicated, using selective serotonin reuptake inhibitors (SSRIs).

2. Internet support groups have increased in popularity due to ease of access, 24-hours-a-day support, and anonymity.

3. One-on-one discussion and individual counseling are helpful.

4. Educate survivors with descriptive information about the need for surveillance, follow-up, and discussions about what constitutes recurrence.

5. Provide positive reappraisal and development of cognitive strategies to maximize coping, enhance a sense of mastery over life, and reevaluate priorities for the future.

Family Relationships (Northouse, 1996; Mellon & Northouse, 2001)

- Breast cancer affects the entire family, and family members have a large role in helping other family members to adjust to the impact of the disease.

- Family members are most often identified as the primary source of emotional support for the patient.

- Differences between breast cancer survivors and family members:

  Perceptions of illness and degree of symptoms

  Subjective experiences in feelings and emotional adjustment

  Distress during different phases of the diagnostic, treatment, and survivorship experience

Patterns of communication and information flow (Rees & Barth, 2000)

Perception of threat

- Demands of illness

  Emotional demands, with spouses reporting feelings of shock, fear, sadness, and remorse

  Physical demands, with spouses taking on additional home routines, particularly during recurrence and metastatic disease

  Strain on social demands and interpersonal relationships

  A range of reactions for young and school-age children: mood and self-esteem changes, academic difficulties (e.g., poor concentration and declining academic performance), somatic symptoms (e.g., stomachache, appetite changes, and difficulty sleeping), and social and interpersonal changes (e.g., acting out, withdrawal, and loss of interest).

- Factors in helping families to adjust (Shands, et al., 2000):

  Foster contact and communication with family members who may often feel neglected.

  Family-focused assessment that is not cumbersome; start with a few pointed questions about how the family is adjusting.

  Provide direct information to both patient and family.

Workplace Issues (Hoffman, 1999; Loerzel, 2004)

- Employment and work are important aspects of survivorship.

- Going to work enhances a sense of normalcy and provides social support.

- Some people may feel stigmatized when they return to work. However, federal laws prohibit work discrimination based on cancer history.

- One large study of over 4,000 cancer survivors concerns about work conducted by Schultz and colleagues (2002) found that the majority of cancer survivors did not perceive employment-related problems and were assimilated back into the work force. However:

  8.5% were unable to work

  7.3% experienced job discrimination

  Age, gender, ethnic group, and cancer type affected working status of survivors

- Suggestions to help breast cancer survivors return to work.

  1. Carefully assess fatigue, cognitive changes, and other side effects after treatment that may affect one's return to work full time.

  2. Assess the feasibility of the return to full-time work. Consider a plan for a gradual increase in work time.

  3. Privacy issues are very important. One does not have to disclose one's cancer history unless it directly affects one's work performance.

4. Take stock of insurance, reimbursement, and other benefits that may be affected by cancer history.

Internet Cancer Support Groups (Schmidt & Andrykowski, 2004; Eysenbach, 2003; Hoybye, et al., 2004)

-   The Internet is increasingly used as a means of support for cancer survivors.

-   Estimates are that about 39% of persons with cancer use the Internet.

-   The Internet support helps to decrease social isolation and can aid as a good method for cancer rehabilitation.

Meaning and Purpose in Life (Dow, et al., 1999; Utley, 1999; Taylor, 2000)

-   The search for meaning is a basic human need; one that is necessary for human fulfillment.

-   Deriving meaning in life is often postponed until such time that individuals face their own mortality, experience suffering, or undergo a life-changing experience, such as cancer.

-   The process of making meaning from a cancer experience may include finding a causal attribution, finding the silver lining in the experience of suffering, making downward social comparisons, searching for a higher order in the experience, and placing the cancer experience within the larger context of one's life.

- The process of making meaning occurs over time, and the means by which one derives meaning are diverse. They may include support group activities, individual counseling, keeping a journal, advocacy and activism, and volunteerism.

- Positive outcomes of making meaning are increased coping, hopefulness, and transcendence.

- Meaning of cancer survivorship themes were derived from the study of cancer survivors (Dow, et al., 1999).

  Having a balance between the experience of increased dependence while seeking independence and interdependence

  Seeking a sense of wholeness after a life-changing experience

  Facing the challenge of putting the cancer experience within the context of one's life

  Struggling between elements of basic survival and reclaiming one's life

  Managing physical symptoms that persist and linger over the long term

  Facing multiple losses

  Gaining a sense of control rather than being controlled

  Contrasting the focus between seizing the day and looking to the future

- Management:

  1. Recognition and support for spiritual needs may fluctuate over time.

  2. Maintain hope despite advancing disease.

RESOURCES

- American Cancer Society: Cancer Survivors' Network at http://cancersurvivorsnetwork.org
- Breast Cancer Survivors Network at www.bcsn.org

REFERENCES

Badger, T., Segrin, C., Meek, P., Lopez, A. M., & Bonham, E. (2004). A case study of telephone interpersonal counseling for women with breast cancer and their partners. *Oncology Nursing Forum, 31*(5), 997–1003.

Bennett, B., Goldstein, D., Lloyd, A., Davenport, T., & Hickie, I. (2004). Fatigue and psychological distress—Exploring the relationship in women treated for breast cancer. *European Journal of Cancer, 40*(11), 1689–1695.

Brandt, B. (1996). Depression in women with breast cancer. In K. H. Dow (Ed.), *Contempory issues in breast cancer* (pp. 107–120). Sudbury, MA: Jones & Bartlett.

Clark, E. J., Stovall, E. L., Leigh, S., Siu, A. L., Austin, D. K., & Rowland, J. H. (1996). *Imperatives for quality cancer care: Access advocacy, action and accountability*. Silver Springs, MD: National Coalition for Cancer Survivorship.

Dow, K. H., Ferrel, B. R., Haberman, M. R., & Eaton, L. (1999). The meaning of quality of life in cancer survivorship. *Oncology Nursing Forum, 26*, 519–528.

Dow, K. H., Ferrell, B. R., Leigh, S., Ly, J., & Gulasekaram, P. (1996). An evaluation of the quality of life in long-term breast cancer survivors. *Breast Cancer Research and Treatment, 39*, 261–273.

Eysenbach, G. (2003). The impact of the Internet on cancer outcomes. *CA: A Cancer Journals for Clinicians, 53*(6), 356–371.

Frost, M. H., Arvizu, R. D., Jayakumar, S., Schoonover, A., Novotny, P., & Zahasky, K. (1999). A multidisciplinary healthcare delivery model for women with breast cancer: Patient satisfaction and physical and psychosocial adjustment. *Oncology Nursing Forum, 26*(10), 1673–1680.

Gobel, B. (2000). Anxiety. In C. H. Yarbro, M. H. Frogge, & M. Goodman (Eds.), *Cancer symptom management* (2nd ed., pp. 580–590). Sudbury, MA: Jones & Bartlett.

Hoffman, B. (1999). Cancer survivors' employment and insurance rights: A primer for oncologists. *Oncology (Huntingt), 13*(6), 841–846; discussion 846, 849, 852.

Hoybye, M. T., Johansen, C., & Tjornhoj-Thomsen, T. (2004). Online interaction. Effects of storytelling in an Internet breast cancer support group. *Psychooncology 14*(3): 211–220.

Lehto, R. H., & Cimprich, B. (1999). Anxiety and directed attention in women awaiting breast cancer surgery. *Oncology Nursing Forum, 26*(4), 767–772.

Loerzel, V. W. (2004). Support and survivorship issues. In K. H. Dow (Ed.), *Contemporary issues in breast cancer: A nursing persective* (2nd ed., pp. 313–321). Sudbury, MA: Jones & Bartlett.

Love, A. W., Grabsch, B., Clarke, D. M., Bloch, S., & Kissane, D. W. (2004). Screening for depression in women with metastatic breast cancer: A comparison of the Beck Depression Inventory Short Form and the Hospital Anxiety and Depression Scale. *Australian and New Zealand Journal of Psychiatry, 38*(7), 526–531.

McDonald, M. V., Passik, S. D., Dugan, W., Rosenfeld, B., Theobald, D. E., & Edgerton, S. (1999). Nurses' recognition of depression in their patients with cancer. *Oncology Nursing Forum, 26*(3), 593–599.

Mellon, S., & Northouse, L. L. (2001). Family survivorship and quality of life following a cancer diagnosis. *Research in Nursing & Health, 24*(6), 446–459.

Montazeri, A., Sajadian, A., Ebrahimi, M., & Akbari, M. E. (2004). Depression and the use of complementary medicine among breast cancer patients. *Support Care in Cancer*. Retrieved Feb 23, 2005, from www.springerlink.com

Northouse, L. (1996). Spouse and family issues in breast cancer. In K. H. Dow (Ed.), *Contemporary issues in breast cancer* (pp. 163–171). Sudbury, MA: Jones & Bartlett.

Rees, C. E., & Barth, P. (2000). Exploring the information flow: Partners of women with breast cancer, patients, and healthcare professionals. *Oncology Nursing Forum, 27*, 1267–1275.

Ritz, L. J., Nissen, M. J., Swenson, K. K., Farrell, J. B., Sperduto, P. W., Sladek, M. L., et al. (2000). Effects of advanced nursing care on quality of life and cost outcomes of women diagnosed with breast cancer. *Oncology Nursing Forum, 27*(6), 923–932.

Schmidt, J. E., & Andrykowski, M. A. (2004). The role of social and dispositional variables associated with emotional processing in adjustment to breast cancer: An Internet-based study. *Health Psychology, 23*(3), 259–266.

Schultz, P. N., Beck, M. L., Stava, C., & Sellin, R. V. (2002). Cancer survivors: Work related issues. *American Association of Occupational Health Nurses, 50*(5), 220–226.

Shands, M. E., Lewis, F. M., & Zahlis, E. H. (2000). Mother and child interactions about the mother's breast cancer: An interview study. *Oncology Nursing Forum, 27*, 77–85.

Spielberger, C., Gorush, R., & Lushene, R. (1983). *Manual for the state-trait anxiety inventory.* Palo Alto, CA: Consulting Psychologists Press.

Stephenson, N. L., Weinrich, S. P., & Tavakoli, A. S. (2000). The effects of foot reflexology on anxiety and pain in patients with breast and lung cancer. *Oncology Nursing Forum, 27*(1), 67–72.

Taylor, E. J. (2000). Transformation of tragedy among women surviving breast cancer. *Oncology Nursing Forum, 27*, 781–788.

Utley, R. (1999). The evolving meaning of cancer for long-term survivors of breast cancer. *Oncology Nursing Forum, 26*(9), 1519–1523.

CHAPTER TWENTY-ONE

End of Life and Palliative Care

Background (Hoyer, 2004)

- Although advances have been made in diagnosis and treatment of breast cancer, an estimated 39,600 women die of the disease each year.

- When patients have advanced disease and metastatic disease, the goal of therapy is not cure, but palliation.

- Palliative care is the standard of care for patients with advanced and metastatic breast cancer and focuses on quality of life, alleviation of distressing symptoms, psychosocial support, and assisting family and friends to cope with death and bereavement.

Palliative Care Trajectory

- According to Brant (1998) and McHale (2002), the palliative care trajectory involves three phases

  1. The active phase focuses on treating the disease to prolong life.

  2. The symptomatic phase focuses on the control of the disease to relieve or palliate distressing symptoms.

  3. The supportive phase focuses on comfort and end-of-life issues. Table 21-1 illustrates the palliative care trajectory.

- A palliative care plan is implemented using information about the extent of metastatic disease.

TABLE 21-1

Palliative Care Trajectory

Active Phase	Symptomatic Phase	Supportive Phase
Halt disease progression	Slow or control disease	Treatment is for symptom management, not tumor effect
Provide aggressive treatment	Relief of tumor-related symptoms	Goal: comfortable death
Tolerate toxicities	Less aggressive treatment	
Goal: prolong life	Therapeutic index: balance between benefit and harm	
	Tolerate fewer toxicities	
	Goal: symptom relief/management	

- Metastatic disease can be categorized into three areas:
  1. Bone metastasis
  2. Visceral metastasis
  3. CNS metastasis

     Metastasis can occur in each of these sites or a combination of sites. Signs and symptoms and interventions for metastasis are listed in Table 21-2.

- End-of-life symptom clusters

  There are several end-of-life symptom clusters that occur with metastatic disease. Most common symptoms occurring at the end of life are pain, delirium dyspnea, anorexia/cachexia, and depression.

  The symptoms, causes, and potential interventions are listed on Table 21-3.

- Pain

  Pain in metastatic disease may result from omatic, visceral, and/or neuropathic pain syndromes.

  Somatic pain results primarily from bone metastasis, but may also occur with skin metastasis and lymphedema.

  Visceral pain results from liver metastasis or pleural effusion.

  Neuropathic pain results from CNS metastasis, spinal cord compression, and/or nerve damage.

  Pain management is ongoing and requires regular use of appropriate analgesic and adjuvant drugs.

  In addition, physical therapy and complementary therapy may be used as an adjunct, not substitute, for pharmacologic pain management.

TABLE 21-2
Metastatic Breast Cancer Sites

	Bone	Visceral	CNS
Signs and Symptoms	Pain Pathologic fractures Hypercalcemia Nerve compression Decreased mobility	Depends on site Dyspnea Nausea Abdominal pain Anorexia Constipation	Changes in mental status Confusion Motor disturbances
Interventions	Pain medications Radiation Bisphosphonates Surgery Endocrine therapy Systemic chemotherapy	Systemic chemotherapy Endocrine therapy Symptom relief	Corticosteroids Cranial radiation Intrathecal chemotherapy

TABLE 21-3
End-of-Life Symptom Clusters

Symptoms	Causes	Interventions
Pain	Bone metastases Nerve impingement Tumor pressure Organ obstruction Preexisting chronic pain Depression	Opioids/analgesics Adjuvant medications Physical therapy Complementary and alternative therapies
Delirium	Confusion Hallucinations Sedation Seizures Electrolyte imbalances Medications CNS metastases Sleep disturbances	Haloperidol Chlorpromazine Oxygen therapy Terminal sedation
Dyspnea	Visceral metastases Anemia Serous effusions	Oxygen therapy Nebulizer Diuretics Treatment of effusions Scopolamine patches
Anorexia/ cachexia	Xerostomia Taste changes Tumor effects Constipation Nausea Bowel obstruction	Mouth moisturizers/ oral care Small, frequent meals Laxatives Antiemetic therapies
Depression	Social withdrawal Sleep changes Weight loss Suicidal ideation Hopelessness	Antidepressants Support groups Counseling or psychotherapy

- Delirium

    Delirium is often more distressing to the family rather than to the patient.

    Patients may be disoriented, agitated, restless, and have memory loss, confusion, change in sleep patterns, and general impairment of cognitive function.

    Delirium may be associated with opioid use, CNS metastasis, hepatic encephalopathy, and dyspnea.

    Thus, the causative factors of delirium must be identified and appropriate treatment instituted.

    At the end of life, treatment of delirium has been haloperidol .5–2.0 mg every 4 to 6 hours.

- Effusion

    Pleural, pericardial, and abdominal effusions occur with metastatic breast cancer.

    Accompanying symptoms include dyspnea, fatigue, tachycardia, anorexia, confusion, restlessness, constipation, and early satiety.

    Symptom management of pleural effusion, the most common effusion, has been a combination of oxygen therapy, nebulizer, diuretics, opiates, and scopolamine patches to manage secretions.

    Symptom management for pericardial effusion may be pericardiocentesis.

    Symptom management for ascites is peritoneal catheter to promote comfort and increase drainage.

- Anorexia and cachexia

    The etiology of anorexia and cachexia is not well understood.

    Megestrol acetate has been used to stimulate appetite and weight gain in advanced disease. However, performance status and quality of life have not been affected by this drug (Vadell, et al., 1998).

    When death is imminent, there is a decreased need for food and fluid.

    Teaching and support are directed to the family to understand that food and hydration may prolong patient suffering.

- Communication at end of life

    Communication and decision making are particularly complex at the end of life.

    Conflicts can arise when the patient and family are at odds as to whether the decision is to continue or to end treatment.

    Clarification of patient wishes and support for decision making are very critical.

REFERENCES

Brant, J. M. (1998). The art of palliative care: Living with hope, dying with dignity. *Oncology Nursing Forum, 25*(6), 995–1004.

Hoyer, K. (2004). End of life and palliative care. In K. H. Dow (Ed.), *Contemporary issues in breast cancer: A nursing persective* (2nd ed., pp. 323–333). Sudbury, MA: Jones & Bartlett.

McHale, H. K. (2002). Palliative care. In K. Kuebler & P. Esper (Eds.), *Palliative practices from A–Z* (pp. 193–197). Pittsburgh, PA: Oncology Nursing Society.

Vadell, C., Segui, M. A., Gimenez-Arnau, J. M., Morales, S., Cirera, L., Bestit, I., et al. (1998). Anticachectic efficacy of megestrol acetate at different doses and versus placebo in patients with neoplastic cachexia. *American Journal of Clinical Oncology, 21*(4), 347–351.

Index

NOTE: Page numbers with *f* refer to figures, with *t* to tables.